A Mental Health Provider's Guide to Telehealth

This book works as a guide to videoconferencing practice for psychological providers through a broad, simplified, and practical overview of pertinent factors. It is a consolidation of research literature and professional experiences of practicing, teaching, and studying videoconferencing.

It begins by defining key concepts such as telehealth, telepsychology, and other related terminology and examining the role of telehealth in addressing ongoing mental health disparities. An overview of existing videoconferencing practices, guidebooks and general recommendations, as well as specifics of ethical and legal factors are discussed. The book then details numerous essential factors of videoconferencing practice that are directly applicable to psychological care, including considerations of computer system, video camera, display screen, microphone, videoconferencing platform, bandwidth and latency, and room setup, along with self-care practices. The appendices provide readers with links to resources, checklists, and other documents to guide their practice.

Psychologists, counselors, and other mental health providers will find this user-friendly, research-informed guide indispensable when implementing online treatment and teletherapy.

Jonathan G. Perle, PhD, ABPP, is a board-certified clinical child and adolescent psychologist and educator. He has significant experience related to the study, teaching, and utilization of telehealth modalities.

T0373552

A Mental Health Provider's Guide to Telehealth

Providing Outpatient Videoconferencing Services

Jonathan G. Perle

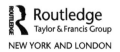

NEW YORK AND LONDON

First published 2021
by Routledge
605 Third Avenue, New York, NY 10158

and by Routledge
2 Park Square, Milton Park, Abingdon, Oxon OX14 4RN

Routledge is an imprint of the Taylor & Francis Group, an informa business

Library of Congress Cataloging-in-Publication Data
Names: Perle, Jonathan, author.
Title: A mental health provider's guide to telehealth: providing
outpatient videoconferencing services / Jonathan Perle.
Description: New York, NY: Routledge, 2021. |
Includes bibliographical references and index.
Identifiers: LCCN 2020045880 (print) | LCCN 2020045881 (ebook) |
ISBN 9780367713591 (hardback) | ISBN 9780367713577 (paperback) |
ISBN 9781003150473 (ebook)
Subjects: LCSH: Mental health services–Computer network resources. |
Videoconferencing. | Telecommunication in medicine.
Classification: LCC RA790.5 .P43 2021 (print) |
LCC RA790.5 (ebook) | DDC 610.285–dc23
LC record available at https://lccn.loc.gov/2020045880
LC ebook record available at https://lccn.loc.gov/2020045881

ISBN: 978-0-367-71359-1 (hbk)
ISBN: 978-0-367-71357-7 (pbk)
ISBN: 978-1-003-15047-3 (ebk)

Typeset in Times New Roman
by Newgen Publishing UK

Contents

Figures

Tables

Author Biography

Jonathan G. Perle, PhD, ABPP, is a board-certified clinical child and adolescent psychologist, and assistant professor of clinical psychology. He has significant experience providing clinical assessment and interventions within diverse clinical settings (e.g., medical centers, primary care, schools, university clinics) and roles (e.g., interdisciplinary, multidisciplinary, outpatient, inpatient). In addition to his current responsibilities that include teaching, supervising, mentoring, and conducting research, Dr. Perle provides both face-to-face and virtual psychological care. Beginning in his graduate education and spanning his ongoing career, Dr. Perle has studied, written about, and taught about telehealth modalities. Combined works have resulted in multiple peer-reviewed publications, articles in national periodicals, professional presentations, collaborative projects, consultative services, and his design and implementation of one of the first recognized telehealth-specific doctoral-level courses for clinical psychology students. Dr. Perle has also been recognized as a psychological innovator by the American Psychological Association's *Monitor* for his work designing an evidence-based and Health Insurance Portability and Accountability Act (HIPAA-) compliant smartphone application related to parent management training. In addition to serving as a reviewer for multiple journals, he serves as an editorial board member for the *Journal of Technology in Behavioral Sciences*.

Preface

Purpose and Outline of This Book

The information presented in this book is a collection of research literature, combined with professional experiences related to practicing, teaching about, and studying videoconferencing. The purpose is not to detail every possible aspect of videoconferencing practice, nor provide a long or complicated academic discussion, although research is certainly cited. Rather, this book is designed to guide videoconferencing practice for psychological providers through a broad, simplified, and practical overview of pertinent factors, presented through relatively brief chapters. Of note, while information is generally tailored for the United States and mental health providers, due to the universality of technology much of the applied information can be viewed as applicable to a wider audience.

The book begins with a broad overview defining telehealth, telepsychology, and associated terminology (Chapter 1). Chapter 2 details the research indicating telepsychology, with a focus on videoconferencing, as a viable means of addressing ongoing mental health disparity among those who require psychological healthcare, and those who receive it. To inform ethical and legal practice, Chapter 3 broadly details available guidebooks and recommendation documentation. Recommendations are then consolidated within Chapter 4 through a detailed discussion of specific ethical and legal factors that providers should consider when conducting videoconferencing services. Chapter 5 provides a brief overview of videoconferencing logistics that providers should consider when implementing videoconferencing into their practices. Each item presented in the overview is then detailed in the subsequent Chapters 6 through 14. More specifically, items include discussions of both the provider's and patient's computer systems (Chapter 6), video camera considerations (Chapter 7), display screen considerations (Chapter 8), microphone considerations (Chapter 9), videoconferencing platform considerations (Chapter 10), bandwidth and latency considerations (Chapter 11), room setup considerations (Chapter 12), and finally, video- (Chapter 13), and audio-related tips (Chapter 14). Chapter 15 then details how to document the videoconferencing session content, with discussions of general documentation methods, as well as specifics that can be tailored for initial visits and assessment sessions. To bring together all of the information, Chapter 16 presents brief stepwise lists of setting up and actually conducting the sessions. As increased usage of technology has the potential to create a range of novel physical and ocular challenges, Chapter 17 details self-care practices that providers can adopt to ensure a productive and healthy videoconferencing-based or videoconferencing-enhanced practice. As unique issues may arise (e.g., how to stay up to date, how to engage children or older adults), Chapter 18 presents common questions and answers related to videoconferencing practice. Finally, Chapter 19 closes with a conclusion and recommendations for next steps for providers. In supplement to primary discussions, several appendices are also provided. Appendices include acronyms used in this book (Appendix A), definitions related to the videoconferencing practices (Appendix B), a consolidated listing of formal guidelines and recommendation documentation to guide practice (Appendix C), a consolidated listing of helpful resources related to videoconferencing (Appendix D), a consolidated listing of general organizations that providers should review and consider following for ongoing information (Appendix E), a consolidated listing of helpful books and journals that frequently publish mental health-focused telehealth information (Appendix F), a list of possible continuing education programming for providers who desire more training (Appendix G), a summarized overview of the entire videoconferencing practice for providers (Appendix H), a comprehensive videoconferencing provider checklist (Appendix I), a simplified and brief provider checklist (Appendix J), videoconferencing coloring pages that providers may employ to normalize the videoconferencing process for children (Appendix K), and finally, a patient handout detailing methods of preparing for the videoconferencing sessions (Appendix L). I truly hope that you find the information helpful in your practice!

Disclaimer for Discussions Throughout This Book

While attempts were made to provide an up-to-date discussion of videoconferencing practices for providers, it should be noted that the field of telehealth is a very broad and rapidly developing field. As such, several items should be highlighted. First, while the subject matter is believed to help one begin and maintain a videoconferencing practice, in line with the book's aim to provide a broad, simplified, and practical overview, it is not all encompassing or completely exhaustive, as individual-related issues may arise requiring tailoring of the presented information to ensure a fit for one's practice. Further, while information regarding ethical and legal factors are reviewed, due to the rules being ever evolving, the discussions are meant to provide information and are not meant to act as legal advice. As such, it is suggested that providers seek additional consultation, supervision, and training to ensure that they have proper knowledge to ensure the highest level of both ethical and legal care for their patients. As part of this process, it is suggested that providers (especially those who wish to practice cross-state or cross-country) check with governing bodies to ensure compliance with more specific jurisdictional rules, as well as to monitor for changes that can affect practice. Finally, while examples of products useful for videoconferencing services are presented within the book, their inclusion is for informational purposes. The author is not endorsing one product over the other.

Acknowledgments

I would like to thank several people who have either directly or indirectly supported this work. First, I would like to thank my wife, Alexandria, who has not only been supportive of my writing, but helped contribute through her creation of children's coloring pages that are presented in the appendices. I would also like to thank my dogs, Ripley and Leela, and rabbit, Inky, for providing some much-needed entertainment while writing, as well as posing for some of the images presented in this book. Further, I would like to thank my parents, Eric and Holly, for providing me with the tools to be successful in my professional career. Similarly, a special thank you to Dr. Barry Nierenberg who served as my clinical and academic mentor throughout graduate school. Without his support and assistance throughout my graduate training, I likely would have not been able to pursue a line of work and study related to telehealth. Additionally, a thanks to Robert Allred for taking the time to discuss my ideas and providing feedback on an early draft. Finally, I would like to thank each and every person who purchases this book. I am truly appreciative and hope you find the content relevant and useful in your practice.

1 Defining Telehealth, Telepsychology, and Associated Terms

While the term has become ingrained into society over the last decade as an alternative or supplement to face-to-face (F2F) services, the verbiage used to describe "telehealth" is far from simple. If one were to review peer-reviewed research articles, books, documentation from guiding organizations, and findings from a basic internet search, they would encounter dozens of terms used to describe telehealth processes, as well as a range of associated definitions that vary in detail and focus.

Historical Variability in the Terminology of Telehealth

To account for the uses of technology in healthcare services, numerous terms and phrases have been created (Table 1.1). From the literature, the majority of terms can be grouped into those using prefixes of either "internet-," "e-," or "tele-." For example, "internet therapy," "e-therapy," and "teletherapy" often similarly and broadly refer to the process of providing therapy services through a digital medium. These terms are further supplemented with "online therapy," "distance therapy," and "web therapy." As illustrated by this example, many terms exist to describe similar constructs, with the terms often being used interchangeably within the literature. Potentially due to this inconsistency, no universal nomenclature exists. Nevertheless, the most contemporarily accepted term to describe the integration of technology with healthcare services is simply "telehealth."

Historical Challenges with Defining Telehealth

Even though the name "telehealth" has become increasingly accepted over time, the defining of the term has evidenced additional variability. More specifically, due to so many organizations and researchers attempting to provide a definition, a multitude of variations has ensued, including those proposed by the World Health Organization (WHO, n.d.), Health Resources and Services Administration (HRSA, 2019), Military Health System (MHS, n.d.), US Department of Veterans Affairs (VA, n.d.), American Psychological Association (APA, 2013), American Medical Association (AMA, 2020), American Counseling Association (ACA,

Table 1.1 Mental health-focused telehealth verbiage

Tele-	e-	Internet-	Other
Telehealth	e-therapy	Internet therapy	Behavioral telehealth
Telepsychology	e-health	Internet interventions	Online therapy
Telepsychiatry	e-psychology	Internet-delivered CBT	Distance counseling
Telebehavioral health		Internet-delivered care	Distance therapy
Teletherapy			Web psychology
Telemedicine			Web therapy
Telecare			Digital therapy
			Digital interventions

n.d.), National Association of Social Workers (NASW; Felton, 2020), the American Telemedicine Association (ATA, n.d.), and countless others (Table 1.2). The nonuniversality of what encompasses telehealth has created challenges for researchers and providers to identify and understand what guiding information is available. Unfortunately, such confusion has persisted across considerable time. For example, Baker and Bufka (2011, p. 405) wrote, "A review of relevant state and federal laws reveals inconsistencies even in the terminology used to describe provision of services via technology with some referring to 'telehealth,' others to 'telemedicine,' and others using additional terms," while in 2018, telehealth guidebooks for billing continue to indicate that, "You may hear [terms such as telehealth, telemedicine, and others] used interchangeably as they are broadly defined as using technology to deliver healthcare from a distance" (Coding Institute, 2018, p. 3).

Current Definition of Telehealth

Despite differences in terminology and definitions, several overlapping principles of telehealth emerge to guide understanding and practice. First, telehealth is an umbrella term encompassing numerous fields of healthcare services. Under this umbrella are specialty areas, including telemedicine (i.e., the integration of technology with medical services) and telepsychology (i.e., the integration of technology with psychological services). Each of these primary specialties can be divided into subspecialties, including medical specialties (e.g., telepsychiatry, teledermatology, telesurgery, teleradiology) and psychological orientations (e.g., cognitive-behavioral therapy [CBT], behavioral, cognitive, psychodynamic). Regardless of the specialty and subspecialty, services can be offered through one of two primary service delivery types: synchronous or asynchronous modalities. Synchronous modalities are defined to include live, back-and-forth communication

Table 1.2 Definitions adopted by organizations

Organization	Definition
American Counseling Association (ACA, n.d.)***	Telebehavioral health, or distance counseling, is the use of a digital platform that provides secure, encrypted, audio-video conferencing to communicate with a client in real time. This does not include nonsynchronous (not real-time) texts, calls, digital chats, emails to and from counselors and their clients.
American Medical Association (AMA, 2020)*	Telehealth includes a variety of tools and platforms that allow clinicians to connect with one another as well as with patients. Telehealth between patients and clinicians is most commonly seen as: 1. *Synchronous*: real-time, audio-video communication that connects physicians and patients in different locations; real-time audio and telephone communication. 2. *Asynchronous*: store-and-forward technologies that collect images and data to be transmitted and interpreted later; remote patient-monitoring tools such as blood-pressure monitors, Bluetooth-enabled digital scales, and other wearable devices that can communicate biometric data for review (which may involve the use of mHealth apps).
American Psychological Association (APA, 2013)**	The provision of psychological services using telecommunication technologies.
American Telemedicine Association (ATA, n.d.)*	Technology-enabled health and care management and delivery systems that extend capacity and access.
Health Resources and Services Administration (HRSA, 2019)*	The use of electronic information and telecommunication technologies to support and promote long-distance clinical healthcare, patient and professional health-related education, public health, and health administration. Technologies include videoconferencing, the Internet, store-and-forward imaging, streaming media, and terrestrial and wireless communications.
Military Health System (MHS, n.d.)*	Telehealth is the use of telecommunications and information technologies to provide health assessment, diagnosis, treatment, consultation, education, and health-related information across distances.
National Association of Social Workers (NASW; Felton, 2020)****	Telemental health is the practice of delivering clinical healthcare services via technology-assisted media or other electronic means between a practitioner and a client who are located in two different locations.

(continued)

Table 1.2 Cont.

Organization	Definition
National Telehealth Policy Resource Center (NTPRC, n.d.)*	Telehealth is a collection of means or methods for enhancing healthcare, public health, and health education delivery and support using telecommunications technologies. Telehealth encompasses a broad variety of technologies and tactics to deliver virtual medical, health, and education services. Telehealth is not a specific service, but a collection of means to enhance care and education delivery.
US Department of Veterans Affairs (VA, n.d.)*	Telehealth increases access to high-quality healthcare services by utilizing information and telecommunication technologies to provide healthcare services when the patient and practitioner are separated by geographical distance. The VA subdefines telehealth modalities as clinical video telehealth, home telehealth, and store-and-forward telehealth.
World Health Organization (WHO, n.d.)*	Delivery of healthcare services, where patients and providers are separated by distance. Telehealth uses information and communication technologies (ICT) for the exchange of information for the diagnosis and treatment of diseases and injuries, research and evaluation, and for the continuing education of health professionals.

Notes: * Defined in documentation as "telehealth."
** Defined in documentation as "telepsychology."
*** Defined in documentation as "telebehavioral health."
**** Defined in documentation as "telemental health."

strategies that allow for real-time communication between a provider and a patient (e.g., telephone, videoconferencing, live messaging programs). Contrastingly, asynchronous modalities, often referred to as "store-and-forward," are defined to include methods providing delayed communication. These modalities store information and forward it at another point in time (e.g., email, delayed messaging or texting programs). The two methods can be used to provide a range of specialized clinical healthcare services, including clinical consultation, assessment, intervention, training, supervision, and data management. Such services can be general or more specific (e.g., forensic, neuropsychology). Further, while each can be completed via traditional technology-based methods (e.g., telephone, videoconferencing, email, messaging programs), each can also be provided via mHealth;

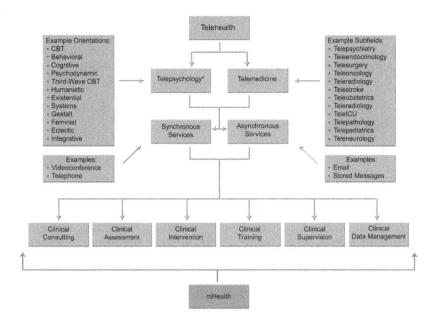

Figure 1.1 Broadly defining telehealth.

Note: * Telemental health and telebehavioral health are often used interchangeably with the term telepsychology.

the integration of mobile technologies with healthcare services (e.g., smartphones, applications [apps]; Perle et al., 2011). See Figure 1.1 for a visual representation of the defining of telehealth services.

Current Definition of Telepsychology

Telepsychology, one of the specialties of telehealth, has vastly expanded over the last decade to encompass a range of synchronous and asynchronous services designed to alleviate symptoms of psychological disorders (Figure 1.2). As adapted from work by Luxton and colleagues (2016, chap. 1), clinical application of telepsychological services can be classified into the six primary categories of: interviews and initial diagnostic meetings, psychological and neuropsychological assessment, psychosocial interventions, data and health-related management among providers, data transmission and monitoring of patients, and professional services.

Interviews and Initial Diagnostic Meetings

Telepsychology has the potential to allow for initial meetings and interviews to be completed from a distance. Such an approach would allow a provider to send diagnostic paperwork via asynchronous methods (e.g., email) before utilizing synchronous modalities to meet a patient or family, introduce the processes of clinical care, review the delivery of telepsychological services, and ultimately conduct the clinical interview in real time via a structured, semi-structured, or unstructured clinical interview. Such information can then be utilized to guide a conceptualization, referrals for additional services or evaluation, and a tailored treatment plan.

Psychological and Neuropsychological Assessment

As based upon diagnostic need, a patient can also complete assessments via telepsychological modalities. Assessments can include basic self-report broadband or narrowband questionnaires, or more complex provider-driven psychological or neuropsychological assessment batteries. For the former, questionnaires could be hosted online if copyright permits, read to the patient over the phone, or viewed by the patient in real time through a provider's screen-sharing program. Further, some assessment companies (e.g., PAR, MHS Assessments, Pearson) have begun creating digital versions of common questionnaires that providers can utilize. Related to formal psychological or neuropsychological assessment batteries, the same companies (e.g., PAR, MHS Assessments, Pearson) have begun hosting paper-based measures for online administration. Further, specific assessments have been either adapted or redeveloped specifically for online administration, complete with digital manipulatives. Further yet, there is ongoing work to create distance-based normative data. To supplement such efforts, several researchers have been actively evaluating which assessments and subscales of the psychological and neuropsychological assessments can be appropriate for online administration and which cannot, given consideration of normative data, potential lag, and the need for manipulatives (e.g., Cullum & Grosch, 2013).

Psychosocial Interventions

Telepsychology also holds the potential for interventions through both synchronous and asynchronous modalities. Such treatments include variations of individual, group, and family therapies for patients across ages, races, ethnicities, and gender identities. Further, they can occur throughout both outpatient and inpatient settings located within medical centers, university clinics, community clinics, correctional facilities, private practices, and schools.

Data and Health-Related Management Among Providers

The technology associated with telepsychology can also assist in the management and communication of clinical data collected as part of the assessment or intervention encounters. More specifically, the proliferation of electronic health records (EHR) not only provided an alternative to paper documentation, but created a less intensive means of transmitting patient information from provider to provider to foster an integrated and team-based approach to patient care. Additionally, the EHR allows a psychological provider to be an active member of the healthcare team through access to information that they may not frequently have an active role in directly assessing, such as medications, vital signs, lab results, and evaluations of physical well-being.

Data Transmission and Monitoring of Patients

Beyond the possibility for data management and communication among healthcare providers, telepsychology also allows for monitoring and communication between the provider and patient, either in a real-time or delayed format. For example, a patient can utilize their smartphone texting feature, or an app, to monitor their mood, anxiety level, or other predetermined factor, with data being transmitted to the provider. While helpful for adults, such strategies can also be used for child patients. For

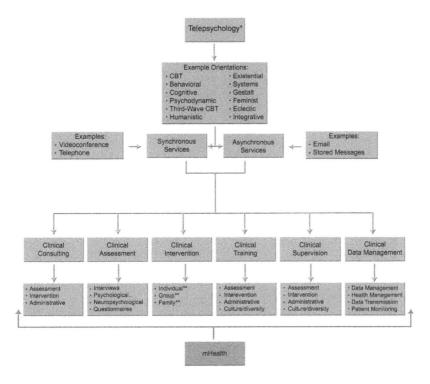

Figure 1.2 Broadly defining telepsychology.

Notes: * Telemental health and telebehavioral health are often used interchangeably with the term telepsychology.

** Outpatient/inpatient.

example, a caregiver could monitor and transmit useful behavioral information to the provider (e.g., frequency of tantrums) to assist in treatment.

Professional Services

Beyond clinical care, telepsychology also provides a wealth of possibilities for professional endeavors. First, the use of technology can allow for distance services, including the possibility for distance consultation about clinical matters, as well as case management. It can also allow for digital meetings and professional presentations on clinical topics. Finally, and of significant interest to many, it can allow for distance teaching and supervision of trainees, both graduate students and those licensed providers looking to become more proficient in specific topics.

Summary Points

- Telehealth has a history of variability of both terminology and definitions.
- Contemporary works suggests that telehealth is an umbrella term that encompasses a range of specialties, such as medical and psychological services. The provision of care can be completed through either synchronous or asynchronous modalities for a range of clinical services, including consultation, assessment, intervention, training, supervision, and data management.
- Telepsychology, a specialization under the telehealth umbrella, refers to the integration of technology with psychological services. Specific services can include the provision of interviews and initial diagnostic meetings, psychological and neuropsychological assessment procedures, psychological interventions, data and health-related management among providers, data transmission and monitoring of patients, and professional services.

References

American Counseling Association (ACA). (n.d.). *Telebehavioral health information and counselors in health care.* Retrieved from www.counseling.org/knowledge-center/mental-health-resources/trauma-disaster/telehealth-information-and-counselors-in-health-care.

American Medical Association (AMA). (2020). *Telehealth implementation playbook.* Retrieved from www.ama-assn.org/system/files/2020-04/ama-telehealth-playbook.pdf.

American Psychological Association (APA). (2013). *Guidelines for the practice of telepsychology.* Retrieved from www.apa.org/practice/guidelines/telepsychology.

American Telemedicine Association (ATA). (n.d.). *Telehealth basics.* Retrieved from www.americantelemed.org/resource/why-telemedicine/.

Baker, D. C., & Bufka, L. F. (2011). Preparing for the telehealth world: Navigating legal, regulatory, reimbursement, and ethical issues in an electronic age. *Professional Psychology: Research and Practice, 42*(6), 405–411. https://doi.org/10.1037/a0025037.

Coding Institute. (2018). *The telemedicine & telehealth handbook for medical practice 2018*. Mountainview, CA: TCI Books.

Cullum, C. M., & Grosch, M. C. (2013). Special considerations in conducting neuropsychology assessment over videoteleconferencing. In K. Myers & C. L. Turvey (Eds.), *Telemental health: Clinical, technical and administrative foundations for evidence-based practice* (pp. 275–290). London: Elsevier.

Felton, E. (2020). Telemental health. National Association of Social Workers. Retrieved from www.socialworkers.org/LinkClick.aspx?fileticket=xmfNHyy8i8M%3D&portalid=0.

Health Resources and Services Administration (HRSA). (2019). *Telehealth programs*. Retrieved from www.hrsa.gov/rural-health/telehealth.

Luxton, D. D., Nelson, E. -L., & Maheu, M. M. (2016). *A practitioner's guide to telemental health: How to conduct legal, ethical and evidence-based telepractice*. Washington, DC: American Psychological Association.

Military Health System (MHS) (n.d.). *Telehealth*. Retrieved from www.health.mil/About-MHS/OASDHA/Defense-Health-Agency/Operations/Clinical-Support-Division/Connected-Health/Telehealth.

National Telehealth Policy Resource Center – Center for Connected Health Policy. (n.d.). About telehealth. Retrieved from www.cchpca.org/about/about-telehealth.

Perle, J. G., Langsam, L. C., & Nierenberg, B. (2011). Controversy clarified: An updated review of clinical psychology and tele-health. *Clinical Psychology Review, 31*(8), 1247–1258. https://doi.org/10.1016/j.cpr.2011.08.003.

US Department of Veterans Affairs (VA). (n.d.). *VA telehealth services*. Retrieved from www.va.gov/anywheretoanywhere/docs/Telehealth_Services_factsheet.PDF.

World Health Organization (WHO). (n.d.). *Telehealth*. Retrieved from www.who.int/gho/goe/telehealth/en/.

2 Mental Health Disparity and the Utility of Videoconferencing Telepsychology

Despite the increasing expansion and popularity of telepsychology, the idea of utilizing technology to assess and treat patients is not a novel notion. What started as a general suggestion of how to address mental health disparity within the literature evolved into a full interest among guiding organizations, clinicians, and researchers. This interest fostered the design, study, and implementation of what would become today's telepsychology practices.

The Ongoing Disparity of Psychological Care

Mental health is one of the largest contributors to worldwide disability, persisting as a challenge for a large portion of the US population (NIMH, 2019; WHO, 2019). Among numerous potential ailments, common psychological diagnoses include anxiety, mood, obsessive-compulsive, trauma-related, psychotic-based, substance use, eating, personality, behavior, and neurodevelopmental disorders. Estimates from 2017 concluded that a general psychological condition, such as noted diagnoses, affects one in five adults. This figure was estimated to represent approximately 18.9 percent of all American adults, equating to 46.6 million individuals 18 years or older (NIMH, 2019). Such numbers are compounded by findings suggesting that approximately one in every four or five youths in the United States may meet criteria for a severely impairing psychological disorder across their lifetime (Merikangas et al., 2010). While varying in degree, psychological diagnoses have been suggested as pervasive across sexes, ages, races, ethnicities, and socioeconomic status (SES; Eaton et al., 2010; NIMH, 2019; Rosenfield & Smith, 2010). If left unaddressed, such challenges have the potential to cause social, occupational, familial, and financial hardships both in the immediate and long term.

While many efficacious (i.e., in controlled research circumstances) and effective (i.e., in real-life circumstances) mental health-focused assessments and treatments have been established to address psychological issues, the reach of providers has historically remained limited. For example, throughout the 2000s, approximately one in five counties within the United States was identified as having an unmet need for psychological providers, with 77 percent of US counties having a shortage of both prescribing and nonprescribing providers (Thomas et al., 2009). As documented by several researchers, disparity has only continued over time (Cook et al., 2017; Whitney & Peterson, 2019).

Internet-Based Telepsychology to Address Mental Health Disparity

Given the substantial need for the expansion of psychological care, the question shifts from "Is there a need?" to "How do we address the need?" One of the most commonly suggested and realistic means of addressing the disparity involves the use of telepsychology. While once deemed logistically impossible due to technological limitations (e.g., too expensive, poor internet connections), the world has changed, with technological evolution creating cheaper, smaller, more powerful, and subsequently more readily available technology for the average person. One of the most important technological developments leading to telepsychology's utility was that of readily available internet. As estimated by the Internet World Stats group (2020), North America saw a 200 percent increase in availability and usage between 2000 and 2020. This rapid increase has led to more individuals within the United States having internet access than those that do not. For example, only an estimated 10 percent of Americans in 2019 had been suggested to not actively utilize the Internet (Anderson et al., 2019). Equally as important, usage has been found to be predominantly ubiquitous across sexes, technology type (e.g., cell phone, desktop computer, laptop, tablet), SES (e.g., some have indicated that lower SES are among the largest adopters of internet-ready smartphones), and ages, including the 65+ age bracket that has shown one of the largest increases among ages (Fjeldsoe et al., 2009; Hiltin, 2018; Pew Research Center, 2017a, 2017b). Finally, there is continued work to provide infrastructure to allow for broadband internet to all locations throughout the United States (Maheu, 2020). Broadband refers to a form of "always on" high-speed internet access that encompasses several types of technologies including fiber optics, wireless, cable, satellite, and digital subscriber line (DSL) (Federal Communications Commission [FCC], 2014). Broadband technologies are common to cities and suburban areas, and are becoming more available in rural areas, allowing for high-speed telepsychological services.

The Advent of Videoconferencing for Mental Healthcare

Due to increases in technology availability and usage, as well as growing recognition that approximately 80 percent of internet users search for healthcare information online (Fox & Duggan, 2013), providers have increasingly recognized the utility of internet-delivered telepsychology to reach those in need. This interest was bolstered by the 2009 signing of the Health Information Technology for Economic and Clinical Health

(HITECH) Act, promoting not only telehealth service utilization, but ongoing study of the mediums (US Department of Health and Human Services [HHS], 2017). While several synchronous and asynchronous telepsychological modalities have been utilized and evaluated, one of the most well-studied, well-supported, and increasingly utilized methods is videoconferencing.

Videoconferencing has risen to the top of possible telepsychology options for both assessment and intervention for several reasons (Table 2.1). First, one of the most cited reasons is the ability to reach populations that are unable to attend F2F services and would otherwise go without psychological care, potentially leading to either the exacerbation of current issues, or the potential development of other comorbid challenges. This inability to attend F2F care may be due to several reasons. Some patients may merely live in areas devoid of providers, such as small towns or rural locations (Bischoff et al., 2004). Due to their physical location, traveling significant distance to a F2F provider in another town may be unreasonable when factoring in potential academic, occupational, or familial demands they may have. Further, this travel can become costly (e.g., gas, parking), especially for patients on a financial budget. Nevertheless, should the patient require general psychological services, or care requiring more specialized knowledge (e.g., specialized experience with rare or complex conditions, providers knowledgeable of unique cultural values), videoconferencing offers the potential to reach the patient where they are (Martinez & Perle, 2019).

Of note, while a large portion of the literature recognizes the importance of videoconferencing for rural healthcare, some have argued that similar rationales relating to transportation and the availability of providers can also apply to urban areas (Perle & Nierenberg, 2013). For example, densely populated cities often have an abundance of psychological providers; however, these providers may predominantly be located outside of the more underserved areas. Further, even for patients who may live within a relatively close proximity to the providers, F2F attendance may still be challenging. To illustrate this point, consider two scenarios. First, consider a single parent who is working full-time and supporting two children. To attend F2F services in a large city, they may have to either arrange for time off from work, or find childcare, both of which could impact finances. Further, due to their work role, the best times for them to attend sessions is unfortunately during rush hour when everyone else is attempting to get out of work. This means that if they are driving to the provider, it could take over one hour each way, creating a three-hour window of when they leave to when they arrive home to their children. This is further complicated by the potential costs of gas and having to park at office buildings, further cutting into finances. Even if they take public transportation, they must still arrange time off from work or for childcare, and hope that the public transportation is running on time. Assuming it is running promptly, this scenario still takes considerable time to get to and from the provider's office. Now, consider a second scenario in which an adult is a caregiver of a child or adult patient with physical disabilities creating mobility issues. Getting the patient to the provider's office could take several hours including the potential loading and unloading of wheelchairs, getting the patient into and out of cars, and arranging care for any other family members that may require assistance (e.g., children). Similar to the first scenario, this all creates time and financial considerations, especially if the psychological care is to be weekly. Unfortunately, these scenarios are not only common, but often prevent even the best-intentioned people from consistently attending therapy. As videoconferencing allows for the patient to be seen in a more convenient location that can reduce time constraints and costs, it can be viewed as very attractive for many providers and patients.

Videoconferencing may also be helpful for those who are not fully open to psychological services. For example, many have documented how some patients oppose and avoid psychological care due to social stigma of what others will think of them (e.g., "I am weak," "I shouldn't need help"; Childress, 2000; Perle et al., 2011). As such, instead of attending F2F, which could be believed by the patient as increasing the chances of someone recognizing them attending the services, videoconferencing can provide a method for the patient to "get their feet wet" with psychological processes in a perceived safe setting. In this regard, the videoconferencing can allow the patient to see what therapy is really like, dispel myths, and potentially lead to them feeling comfortable with pursuing future sessions

Table 2.1 Videoconferencing appropriateness

Helpful for those that:	*Potentially not helpful for those that:*
• Are physically distant from F2F services	• Require more intensive treatments
• Live in rural areas or small towns with limited providers	• Present a serious safety concern to themselves or others
• Have physical disabilities or mobility issues creating issues for transportation	• Do not have a private location to conduct the videoconferencing sessions
• Cannot afford gas for transportation, or parking fees where the provider is located	• Do not have appropriate technology to conduct the videoconferencing sessions
• Need specialized providers	• Utilize deception
• Desire a nonlocal provider due to a small-town social atmosphere	• Are not easily understood
• Need a first step to overcoming stigma	
• Live in urban areas with limited local providers and/or financial, transportation, and/or familial considerations precluding their attendance at F2F care	

either through videoconferencing or F2F. While this notion could apply to anyone who is questioning psychological care, it has been found to be especially pertinent for military personnel (Ben-Zeev et al., 2012), as well as members of specific cultures who may have differing values related to mental health conditions and treatment (e.g., Latinx; Martinez & Perle, 2019).

Research Supporting Videoconferencing Telepsychological Services

While the videoconferencing literature is still considered an emerging field, contemporary research related to psychological care has demonstrated several trends. First, although substantial work focuses on US populations, videoconferencing has been studied and demonstrated to yield positive outcomes internationally, including within Australia (Richardson et al., 2015), China (Poon et al., 2005), Canada (O'Reilly et al., 2007), Spain (De Las Cuevas et al., 2006), and Denmark (Mucic, 2010), among other countries. As based upon such broad evaluation, although not without research demonstrating challenges, if conducted under proper circumstances and with consideration of several unique factors (which will be discussed in detail in later chapters), a significant amount of videoconferencing research has justified its use. For example, providers have been able to effectively conduct clinical interviews (e.g., Bishop et al., 2002), individual therapy (e.g., Berryhill, Halli-Tierney et al., 2019), group therapy (e.g., Frueh et al., 2005; Morland et al., 2004), and family therapy (e.g., Hill et al., 2001) through videoconferencing. Further, while varying by specific measure studied, research has supported the use of videoconferencing administration of specific neuropsychological assessments (Cullum & Grosch, 2013), as well as the Mini Mental Status Examination (Brearly et al., 2017; Cullum & Grosch, 2013; Parikh et al., 2013; Timpano et al., 2013). Combined research for both interventions and assessments has generally demonstrated efficacy and effectiveness for a range of both common and more complex conditions, including mood disorders (Berryhill, Culmer et al., 2019; Osenbach et al., 2013; Varker et al., 2019), anxiety (Berryhill, Halli-Tierney et al., 2019; Varker et al., 2019; Yuen et al., 2013), panic disorder with agoraphobia (Bouchard et al., 2004), eating disorders (Goldfield & Boachie, 2003; Shingleton et al., 2013; Weissman et al., 2020), tic disorders (Himle et al., 2012; Varker et al., 2019), substance-use disorders (Batastini et al., 2016; Lin et al., 2019), obsessive-compulsive disorder (OCD; Goetter et al., 2013; Himle et al., 2006), post-traumatic stress disorder (PTSD; Bolton & Dorstyn, 2015; Lindsay et al., 2015; Olthuis et al., 2016; Varker et al., 2019), adjustment disorder (Varker et al., 2019), suicide prevention (Luxton et al., 2011; Rojas et al., 2019), and behavior disorders involving parent management training (Reese et al., 2015). Further, while limited, some have documented how there is little evidence to support that patients with psychosis have difficulty with videoconferencing or experience an exacerbation of their symptoms (e.g., hallucinations, delusions; Sharp et al., 2011). Perhaps more impressive is the conclusion that videoconferencing interventions and assessments have been successfully applied to children (Duncan et al., 2014; Nelson & Bui, 2010; Nelson et al., 2003; Slone et al., 2012), adults (Backhaus et al., 2012; Varker et al., 2019), and older adults (Egede et al., 2009; Egede et al., 2017; Guilfoyle et al., 2002) across SES, races, sexes, and ethnicities. This remains true both for the general population, and more specialized populations, such as those in the military (Stetz et al., 2013; Waltman et al., 2019), those in forensic and correctional settings (Batastini et al., 2016), and victims of natural disasters (Ruzek et al., 2016).

Of significant importance, while videoconferencing has demonstrated positive outcomes, research has also clarified how such methods correspond to F2F practices. Such evaluation is essential, as even if videoconferencing produces positive results, they may still be inferior to those achieved in F2F interactions. While many documented that initial critics suggested that something would be lost in the videoconferencing process, or that online modalities for serious disorders would not be possible, this has not been proven to be true (Fenichel et al., 2002). Rather, many studies have demonstrated no evidence that psychotherapy provided through videoconferencing is less effective than that provided F2F. This has been concluded as true for a range of conditions including direct treatments for depression (Berryhill, Culmer et al., 2019) and anxiety (Berryhill, Halli-Tierney et al., 2019), as well as for families completing parent management training to address a child's disruptive behavior (Reese et al., 2015).

Positive outcomes comparable with F2F care also apply to the therapeutic alliances that are established throughout the videoconferencing. The general findings show consensus that while there is initial hesitation among both providers and patients towards the use of videoconferencing, following usage, both groups consistently rated moderate to high levels of alliance throughout the therapeutic processes (Kruse et al., 2017; Lozano et al., 2015; Simpson & Reid, 2014). Additionally, many studies have not found major differences in alliance when comparing levels to those achieved in F2F care (Germain et al., 2010; Himle et al., 2012; Jenkins-Guarnieri et al., 2015; Morgan et al., 2008; Simpson, 2001). Simply put, patients will disclose, argue, laugh, and cry as if in a F2F encounter once they become familiar with the videoconferencing methods. Taken together, findings suggest that not only can a strong therapeutic alliance be formed, but it can be sustained. Nevertheless, it should be noted that the research evaluating therapeutic alliance is smaller than other literatures, and mainly comprised of small sample sizes with varied methodologies. Further, not all studies demonstrated equal alliances, as some showed lower levels than F2F treatments (e.g., Greene et al., 2010). As such, while promising, additional research is required to establish more concrete findings, suggesting that those who wish to utilize videoconferencing pay particular attention to their relationships with the patients.

Patient Desire for Videoconferencing Services

Potentially due to increased recognition from the media, increased access to technology, and/or general convenience, both research literature and the general media have documented the increased desire of videoconferencing among patients. For example, large-scale surveys by PwC's Health Research Institute (2015) concluded that over 70 percent of American consumers would utilize telehealth services if given the opportunity. Supplementing general desire, research has also highlighted general satisfaction of videoconferencing following use. More specifically, research has suggested videoconferencing satisfaction across ages and among special populations, such as veterans (Dang et al., 2018; Fletcher et al., 2018; Gros et al., 2018; Jenkins-Guarnieri et al., 2015; Levy et al., 2015; Lindsay et al., 2017; Richardson et al., 2015).

Provider Attitudes Towards Videoconferencing Services

Similar to the patients, providers were initially "lukewarm" when it came to telepsychological services. Despite initial concerns, studies have repeatedly concluded that there remains an interest among many providers for the videoconferencing services (Glueckauf et al., 2018; Perle et al., 2013). Further, although limited research exists to guide conclusions, available studies have documented the generally moderate to high levels of satisfaction of the mediums among providers who have used videoconferencing services (Backhaus et al., 2012; Richardson et al., 2015).

Summary Points

- Mental illness continues to be a serious and ever-increasing challenge.
- Telepsychology proposes a viable and readily available means of addressing disparities to reach the countless in need that go without care.
- While many internet-based telepsychology components are available, videoconferencing has become one of the most well-studied, supported, and popular modalities.
- Telepsychology-focused videoconferencing has demonstrated itself to be an evidence-informed means of fostering positive outcomes for a wide range of mental health difficulties including depression, anxiety, PTSD, panic disorder, eating disorders, tic disorders, substance-use disorders, OCD, adjustment disorders, suicide prevention, and childhood disruptive behavior disorders. Further, it has been generally demonstrated as effective across a range of demographic factors including location, age, sex, and SES.

- Videoconferencing has been evaluated for psychological interviews, individual therapy, group therapy, family therapy, and assessment processes.
- If conducted with consideration of specific factors, videoconferencing has generally produced outcomes equivalent to F2F treatments.
- Available research indicates that a strong therapeutic alliance can be established and maintained through videoconferencing.
- Despite initial hesitations, both patients and providers endorse moderate to high levels of satisfaction with videoconferencing services following use.

References

Anderson, M., Perrin, A., Jiang, J., & Kumar, M. (2019, April 22). 10% of Americans don't use the Internet: Who are they? Pew Research Center. Retrieved from www.pewresearch.org/fact-tank/2019/04/22/some-americans-dont-use-the-internet-who-are-they/.

Backhaus, A., Agha, Z., Maglione, M. L., Repp, A., Ross, B., Zuest, D., ... Thorp, S. R. (2012). Videoconferencing psychotherapy: A systematic review. *Psychological Services*, 9(2), 111–131. https://doi.org/10.1037/a0027924.

Batastini, A. B., King, C. M., Morgan, R. D., & McDaniel, B. (2016). Telepsychological services with criminal justice and substance abuse clients: A systematic review and meta-analysis. *Psychological Services*, 13(1), 20–30. https://doi.org/10.1037/ser0000042.

Ben-Zeev, D., Corrigan, P. W., Britt, T. W., & Langford, L. (2012). Stigma of mental illness and service use in the military. *Journal of Mental Health*, 21(3), 264–273. https://doi.org/10.3109/09638237.2011.621468.

Berryhill, M. B., Culmer, N., Williams, N., Halli-Tierney, A., Betancourt, A., Roberts, H., & King, M. (2019). Videoconferencing psychotherapy and depression: A systematic review. *Telemedicine and e-Health*, 25(6), 435–446. https://doi.org/10.1089/tmj.2018.0058.

Berryhill, M. B., Halli-Tierney, A., Culmer, N., Williams, N., Betancourt, A., King, M., & Ruggles, H. (2019). Videoconferencing psychological therapy and anxiety: A systematic review. *Family Practice*, 36(1), 53–63. https://doi.org/10.1093/fampra/cmy072.

Bischoff, R. J., Hollist, C. S., Smith, C. W., & Flack, P. (2004). Addressing the mental health needs of the rural underserved: Findings from a multiple case study of a behavioral telehealth project. *Contemporary Family Therapy*, 26(2), 179–198. https://doi.org/10.1023/B:COFT.0000031242.83259.fa.

Bishop, J. E., O'Reilly, R. L., Maddox, K., & Hutchinson, L. J. (2002). Client satisfaction in a feasibility study comparing face-to-face interviews with telepsychiatry. *Journal of Telemedicine and Telecare*, 8(4), 217–221. https://doi.org/10.1258/135763302320272185.

Bolton, A. J., & Dorstyn, D. S. (2015). Telepsychology for posttraumatic stress disorder: A systematic review. *Journal of Telemedicine and Telecare*, 21(5), 254–267. https://doi.org/10.1177/1357633X15571996.

Bouchard, S., Paquin, B., Payeur, R., Allard, M., Rivard, V., Fournier, T., ... Lapierre, J. (2004). Delivering cognitive-behavior therapy for panic disorder with agoraphobia in videoconference. *Telemedicine Journal and E-health*, *10*(1), 13–25. https://doi.org/10.1089/153056204773644535.

Brearly, T. W., Shura, R. D., Martindale, S. L., Lazowski, R. A., Luxton, D. D., Shenal, B. V., & Rowland, J. A. (2017). Neuropsychological test administration by videoconference: A systematic review and meta-analysis. *Neuropsychology Review*, *27*(2), 174–186. https://doi.org/10.1007/s11065-017-9349-1.

Childress, C. A. (2000). Ethical issues in providing online psychotherapeutic interventions. *Journal of Medical Internet Research*, *2*(1), e5. https://doi.org/10.2196/jmir.2.1.e5.

Cook, B. L., Trinh, N. H., Li, Z., Hou, S. S. Y., & Progovac, A. M. (2017). Trends in racial-ethnic disparities in access to mental health care, 2004–2012. *Psychiatric Services*, *68*(1), 9–16. https://doi.org/10.1176/appi.ps.201500453.

Cullum, C. M., & Grosch, M. C. (2013). Special considerations in conducting neuropsychology assessment over videoteleconferencing. In K. Myers & C. L. Turvey (Eds.), *Telemental health: Clinical, technical and administrative foundations for evidence-based practice* (pp. 275–290). London: Elsevier.

Dang, S., Gomez-Orozco, C. A., van Zuilen, M. H., & Levis, S. (2018). Providing dementia consultations to veterans using clinical video telehealth: Results from a clinical demonstration project. *Telemedicine and e-Health*, *24*(3), 203–209. https://doi.org/10.1089/tmj.2017.0089.

De Las Cuevas, C. D. L., Arredondo, M. T., Cabrera, M. F., Sulzenbacher, H., & Meise, U. (2006). Randomized clinical trial of telepsychiatry through videoconference versus face-to-face conventional psychiatric treatment. *Telemedicine Journal & e-Health*, *12*(3), 341–350. https://doi.org/10.1089/tmj.2006.12.341.

Duncan, A. B., Velasquez, S. E., & Nelson, E. L. (2014). Using videoconferencing to provide psychological services to rural children and adolescents: A review and case example. *Journal of Clinical Child & Adolescent Psychology*, *43*(1), 115–127. https://doi.org/10.1080/15374416.2013.836452.

Eaton, W. W., Muntaner, C., & Sapag, J. C. (2010). Socioeconomic stratification and mental disorder. In T. L. Scheid & T. N. Brown (Eds.), *A handbook for the study of mental health: Social contexts, theories, and systems* (2nd ed., pp. 226–255). Cambridge, UK: Cambridge University Press.

Egede, L. E., Frueh, C. B., Richardson, L. K., Acierno, R., Mauldin, P. D., Knapp, R. G., & Lejuez, C. (2009). Rationale and design: Telepsychology service delivery for depressed elderly veterans. *Trials*, *10*, 22. https://doi.org/10.1186/1745-6215-10-22.

Egede, L. E., Gebregziabher, M., Walker, R. J., Payne, E. H., Acierno, R., & Frueh, B. C. (2017). Trajectory of cost overtime after psychotherapy for depression in older Veterans via telemedicine. *Journal of Affective Disorders*, *207*, 157–162. https://doi.org/10.1016/j.jad.2016.09.044.

Federal Communications Commission (FCC). (2014, June 23). *Types of broadband connections.* Retrieved from www.fcc.gov/general/types-broadband-connections.

Fenichel, M., Suler, J., Barak, A., Zelvin, E., Jones, G., Munro, K., ... Walker-Schmucker, W. (2002). Myths and realities of online clinical work. *CyberPsychology & Behavior*, *5*(5), 481–497. https://doi.org/10.1089/109493102761022904.

Fjeldsoe, B. S., Marshall, A. L., & Miller, Y. D. (2009). Behavior change interventions delivered by mobile telephone short-message service. *American Journal of Preventative Medicine*, *36*(2), 165–173. https://doi.org/10.1016/j.amepre.2008.09.040.

Fletcher, T. L., Hogan, J. B., Keegan, F., Davis, M. L., Wassef, M., Day, S., & Lindsay, J. A. (2018). Recent advances in delivering mental health treatment via video to home. *Current Psychiatry Reports*, *20*(8), 56. https://doi.org/10.1007/s11920-018-0922-y.

Fox, S., & Duggan, M. (2013, January 15). Health online 2013. Pew Research Center. www.pewresearch.org/internet/2013/01/15/health-online-2013/.

Frueh, B. C., Henderson, S., & Myrick, H. (2005). Telehealth service delivery for persons with alcoholism. *Journal of Telemedicine and Telecare*, *11*(7), 372–375. https://doi.org/10.1177/1357633X0501100701.

Germain, V., Marchand, A., Bouchard, S., Guay, S., & Drouin, M. S. (2010). Assessment of the therapeutic alliance in face-to-face or videoconference treatment for posttraumatic stress disorder. *Cyberpsychology, Behavior, and Social Networking*, *13*(1), 29–35. https://doi.org/10.1089/cyber.2009.0139.

Glueckauf, R. L., Maheu, M. M., Drude, K. P., Wells, B. A., Wang, Y., Gustafson, D. J., & Nelson, E. L. (2018). Survey of psychologists' telebehavioral health practices: Technology use, ethical issues, and training needs. *Professional Psychology: Research and Practice*, *49*(3), 205–219. https://doi.org/10.1037/pro0000188.

Goetter, E. M., Herbert, J. D., Forman, E. M., Yuen, E. K., Gershkovich, M., Glassman, L. H., ... Goldstein, S. P. (2013). Delivering exposure and ritual prevention for obsessive–compulsive disorder via videoconference: Clinical considerations and recommendations. *Journal of Obsessive-Compulsive and Related Disorders*, *2*(2), 137–145. https://doi.org/10.1016/j.jocrd.2013.01.003.

Goldfield, G. S., & Boachie, A. (2003). Case report: Delivery of family therapy in the treatment of anorexia nervosa using telehealth. *Telemedicine Journal and e-Health*, *9*(1), 111–114. https://doi.org/10.1089/153056203763317729.

Greene, C. J., Morland, L. A., Macdonald, A., Frueh, B. C., Grubbs, K. M., & Rosen, C. S. (2010). How does tele-mental health affect group therapy process? Secondary analysis of a noninferiority trial. *Journal of Consulting and Clinical Psychology*, *78*(5), 746–750. https://doi.org/10.1037/a0020158.

Gros, D. F., Lancaster, C. L., López, C. M., & Acierno, R. (2018). Treatment satisfaction of home-based telehealth versus in-person delivery of prolonged exposure for combat-related PTSD in veterans. *Journal of Telemedicine and Telecare*, *24*(1), 51–55. https://doi.org/10.1177/1357633X16671096.

Guilfoyle, C., Wootton, R., Hassall, S., Offer, J., Warren, M., Smith, D., & Eddie, M. (2002). Videoconferencing in facilities providing care for elderly people. *Journal of Telemedicine and Telecare*, *8*(3 suppl.), 22–24. https://doi.org/10.1258/13576330260440745.

Hill, J. V., Allman, L. R., & Ditzler, T. F. (2001). Utility of real-time video teleconferencing in conducting family mental health sessions: Two case reports. *Telemedicine Journal and E-Health*, *7*(1), 55–59. https://doi.org/10.1089/153056201300093930.

Hiltin, P. (2018, September 28). Internet, social media use and device ownership in U.S. have plateaued after years of growth. Pew Research Center. Retrieved from www.pewresearch.org/fact-tank/2018/09/28/internet-social-media-use-and-device-ownership-in-u-s-have-plateaued-after-years-of-growth/.

Himle, J. A., Fischer, D. J., Muroff, J. R., van Etten, M. L., Lokers, L. M., Abelson, J. L., & Hanna, G. L. (2006). Videoconferencing-based cognitive-behavioral therapy for obsessive-compulsive disorder. *Behaviour Research and Therapy*, *44*(12), 1821–1829. https://doi.org/10.1016/j.brat.2005.12.010.

Himle, M. B., Freitag, M., Walther, M., Franklin, S. A., Ely, L., & Woods, D. W. (2012). A randomized pilot trial comparing videoconference versus face-to-face delivery of behavior therapy for childhood tic disorders. *Behaviour Research and Therapy*, *50*(9), 565–570. https://doi.org/10.1016/j.brat.2012.05.009.

Internet World Stats (2020, March 3). Internet users distribution in the world: 2020 Q1. Retrieved from www.internetworldstats.com/stats.htm.

Jenkins-Guarnieri, M. A., Pruitt, L. D., Luxton, D. D., & Johnson, K. (2015). Patient perceptions of telemental health: Systematic review of direct comparisons to in-person psychotherapeutic treatments. *Telemedicine and e-Health*, *21*(8), 652–660. http://dx.doi.org.mwu.idm.oclc.org/10.1089/tmj.2014.0165.

Kruse, C. S., Krowski, N., Rodriguez, B., Tran, L., Vela, J., & Brooks, M. (2017). Telehealth and patient satisfaction: A systematic review and narrative analysis. *BMJ Open*, *7*(8), e016242. http://dx.doi.org/10.1136/bmjopen-2017-016242.

Levy, C. E., Silverman, E., Jia, H., Geiss, M., & Omura, D. (2015). Effects of physical therapy delivery via home video telerehabilitation on functional and health-related quality of life outcomes. *Journal of Rehabilitation Research and Development*, *52*(3), 361–369. https://doi.org/10.1682/JRRD.2014.10.0239.

Lin, L. A., Casteel, D., Shigekawa, E., Weyrich, M. S., Roby, D. H., & McMenamin, S. B. (2019). Telemedicine-delivered treatment interventions for substance use disorders: A systematic review. *Journal of Substance Abuse Treatment*, *101*, 38–49. https://doi.org/10.1016/j.jsat.2019.03.007.

Lindsay, J. A., Hudson, S., Martin, L., Hogan, J. B., Nessim, M., Graves, L., … White, D. (2017). Implementing video to home to increase access to evidence-based psychotherapy for rural veterans. *Journal of Technology in Behavioral Science*, *2*(3–4), 140–148. https://doi.org/10.1007/s41347-017-0032-4.

Lindsay, J. A., Kauth, M. R., Hudson, S., Martin, L. A., Ramsey, D. J., Daily, L., & Rader, J. (2015). Implementation of video telehealth to improve access to evidence-based psychotherapy for posttraumatic stress disorder. *Telemedicine and e-Health*, *21*(6), 467–472. https://doi.org/10.1089/tmj.2014.0114.

Lozano, B. E., Birks, A. H., Kloezeman, K., Cha, N., Morland, L. A., & Tuerk, P. W. (2015). Therapeutic alliance in clinical videoconferencing: Optimizing the communication context. In P. W. Tuerk & P. Shore (Eds.), *Clinical videoconferencing in telehealth: Program development and practice* (pp. 221–251). Cham: Springer International.

Luxton, D. D., June, J. D., & Kinn, J. T. (2011). Technology-based suicide prevention: Current applications and future directions. *Telemedicine and e-Health*, *17*(1), 50–54. https://doi.org/10.1089/tmj.2010.0091.

Maheu, M. M. (2020, July 5). Telehealth reform: U.S. Congress heeds public outcry. Telebehavioral Health Institute. Retrieved from https://telehealth.org/blog/telehealth-reform/#:~:text=July%205%2C%202020-,Telehealth%20Reform%3A%20US%20Congress%20Heeds%20Public%20Outcry,the%20permanent%20expansion%20of%20telehealth.

Martinez, M., & Perle, J. G. (2019). Reaching the Latino population: A brief conceptual discussion on the use of telehealth to address healthcare disparities for the large and growing population. *Journal of Technology in Behavioral Science*, *4*(3), 267–273. https://doi.org/10.1007/s41347-019-00088-9.

Merikangas, K. R., He, J. -P., Burstein, M., Swanson, S. A., Avenevoli, S., Cui, L., … Swendsen, J. (2010). Lifetime prevalence of mental disorders in U.S. adolescents: Results from the National Comorbidity Study – Adolescent

Supplement (NCS-A). *Journal of the American Academy of Child and Adolescent Psychiatry*, *49*(10), 980–989. https://doi.org/10.1016/j.jaac.2010.05.017.

Morgan, R. D., Patrick, A. R., & Magaletta, P. R. (2008). Does the use of telemental health alter the treatment experience? Inmates' perceptions of telemental health versus face-to-face treatment modalities. *Journal of Consulting and Clinical Psychology*, *76*(1), 158–168. https://doi.org/10.1037/0022-006X.76.1.158.

Morland, L. A., Pierce, K., & Wong, M. Y. (2004). Telemedicine and coping skills groups for Pacific Island veterans with post-traumatic stress disorder: A pilot study. *Journal of Telemedicine and Telecare*, *10*(5), 286–289. https://doi.org/10.1258/1357633042026387.

Mucic, D. (2010). Transcultural telepsychiatry and its impact on patient satisfaction. *Journal of Telemedicine and Telecare*, *16*(5), 237–242. https://doi.org/10.1258/jtt.2009.090811.

National Institute of Mental Health (NIMH). (2019, February). Mental illness. Retrieved from www.nimh.nih.gov/health/statistics/mental-illness.shtml.

Nelson, E. -L., Barnard, M., & Cain, S. (2003). Treating childhood depression over videoconferencing. *Telemedicine Journal and E-health*, *9*(1), 49–55. https://doi.org/10.1089/153056203763317648.

Nelson, E. -L., & Bui, T. (2010). Rural telepsychology services for children and adolescents. *Journal of Clinical Psychology*, *66*(5), 490–501. https://doi.org/10.1002/jclp.20682.

O'Reilly, R., Bishop, J., Maddox, K., Hutchinson, L., Fisman, M., & Takhar, J. (2007). Is telepsychiatry equivalent to face-to-face psychiatry? Results from a randomized controlled equivalence trial. *Psychiatric Services*, *58*(6), 836–843. https://doi.org/10.1176/appi.ps.58.6.836.

Olthuis, J. V., Wozney, L., Asmundson, G. J., Cramm, H., Lingley-Pottie, P., & McGrath, P. J. (2016). Distance-delivered interventions for PTSD: A systematic review and meta-analysis. *Journal of Anxiety Disorders*, *44*, 9–26. https://doi.org/10.1016/j.janxdis.2016.09.010.

Osenbach, J. E., O'Brien, K. M., Mishkind, M., & Smolenski, D. J. (2013). Synchronous telehealth technologies in psychotherapy for depression: A meta-analysis. *Depression and Anxiety*, *30*(11), 1058–1067. https://doi.org/10.1002/da.22165.

Parikh, M., Grosch, M. C., Graham, L. L., Hynan, L. S., Weiner, M., Shore, J. H., & Cullum, C. M. (2013). Consumer acceptability of brief videoconference-based neuropsychological assessment in older individuals with and without cognitive impairment. *The Clinical Neuropsychologist*, *27*(5), 808–817. https://doi.org/10.1080/13854046.2013.791723.

Perle, J. G., Langsam, L. C., & Nierenberg, B. (2011). Controversy clarified: An updated review of clinical psychology and tele-health. *Clinical Psychology Review*, *31*(8), 1247–1258. https://doi.org/10.1016/j.cpr.2011.08.003.

Perle, J. G., Langsam, L. C., Randel, A., Lutchman, S., Levine, A. B., Odland, A. P., … Marker, C. D. (2013). Attitudes toward psychological telehealth: Current and future clinical psychologists' opinions of Internet-based interventions. *Journal of Clinical Psychology*, *69*(1), 100–113. https://doi.org/10.1002/jclp.21912.

Perle, J. G., & Nierenberg, B. (2013). How psychological telehealth can alleviate society's mental health burden: A literature review. *Journal of Technology in Human Services*, *31*(1), 22–41. https://doi.org/10.1080/15228835.2012.760332.

Pew Research Center. (2017a, January 11). Internet use by age. Retrieved from www.pewresearch.org/internet/chart/internet-use-by-age/.

Pew Research Center. (2017b, January 11). Internet use by gender. Retrieved from www.pewresearch.org/internet/chart/internet-use-by-gender/.

Poon, P., Hui, E., Dai, D., Kwok, T., & Woo, J. (2005). Cognitive intervention for community-dwelling older persons with memory problems: Telemedicine versus face-to-face treatment. *International Journal of Geriatric Psychiatry*, *20*(3), 285–286. https://doi.org/10.1002/gps.1282.

PwC Health Research Institute (2015). Top health industry issues of 2016: Thriving in the new health economy. Retrieved from www.pwchk.com/en/people-and-organisation/hc-top-issues-dec2015.pdf.

Reese, R. J., Slone, N. C., Soares, N., & Sprang, R. (2015). Using telepsychology to provide a group parenting program: A preliminary evaluation of effectiveness. *Psychological Services*, *12*(3), 274–282. https://doi.org/10.1037/ser0000018.

Richardson, L., Reid, C., & Dziurawiec, S. (2015). "Going the extra mile": Satisfaction and alliance findings from an evaluation of videoconferencing telepsychology in rural western Australia. *Australian Psychologist*, *50*(4), 252–258. https://doi.org/10.1111/ap.12126.

Rojas, S. M., Carter, S. P., McGinn, M. M., & Reger, M. A. (2019). A review of telemental health as a modality to deliver suicide-specific interventions for rural populations. *Telemedicine and e-Health*, *26*(6), 700–709. https://doi.org/10.1089/tmj.2019.0083.

Rosenfield, S., & Smith, D. (2010). Gender and mental health: Do men and women have different amounts or types of problems? In T. L. Scheid & T. N. Brown (Eds.), *A handbook for the study of mental health: Social contexts, theories, and systems* (2nd ed., pp. 226–255). Cambridge, UK: Cambridge University Press.

Ruzek, J. I., Kuhn, E., Jaworski, B. K., Owen, J. E., & Ramsey, K. M. (2016). Mobile mental health interventions following war and disaster. *mHealth*, *2*, 37. https://doi.org/10.21037/mhealth.2016.08.06

Sharp, I. R., Kobak, K. A., & Osman, D. A. (2011). The use of videoconferencing with patients with psychosis: A review of the literature. *Annals of General Psychiatry*, *10*, 14. https://doi.org/10.1186/1744-859X-10-14.

Shingleton, R. M., Richards, L. K., & Thompson-Brenner, H. (2013). Using technology within the treatment of eating disorders: A clinical practice review. *Psychotherapy*, *50*(4), 576–582. https://doi.org/10.1037/a0031815.

Simpson, S. (2001). The provision of a telepsychology service to Shetland: Client and therapist satisfaction and the ability to develop a therapeutic alliance. *Journal of Telemedicine and Telecare*, *7*(1 suppl.), 34–36. https://doi.org/10.1177/1357633X010070S114.

Simpson, S. G., & Reid, C. L. (2014). Therapeutic alliance in videoconferencing psychotherapy: A review. *Australian Journal of Rural Health*, *22*(6), 280–299. https://doi.org/10.1111/ajr.12149.

Slone, N. C., Reese, R. J., & McClellan, M. J. (2012). Telepsychology outcome research with children and adolescents: A review of the literature. *Psychological Services*, *9*(3), 272–292. https://doi.org/10.1037/a0027607.

Stetz, M. C., Folen, R. A., Horn, S. V., Ruseborn, D., & Samuel, K. M. (2013). Technology complementing military psychology programs and services in the Pacific Regional Medical Command. *Psychological Services*, *10*(3), 283–288. https://doi.org/10.1037/a0027896.

Thomas, K. C., Ellis, A. R., Konrad, T. R., Holzer, C. E., & Morrissey, J. P. (2009). County-level estimates of mental health professional shortage in the

United States. *Psychiatric Services, 60*(10), 1323–1328. https://doi.org/10.1176/ps.2009.60.10.1323.

Timpano, F., Pirrotta, F., Bonanno, L., Marino, S., Marra, A., Bramanti, P., & Lanzafame, P. (2013). Videoconference-based mini mental state examination: A validation study. *Telemedicine and e-Health, 19*(12), 931–937. https://doi.org/10.1089/tmj.2013.0035.

US Department of Health and Human Services (HHS). (2017). *HITECH act enforcement interim final rule.* Retrieved from www.hhs.gov/hipaa/for-professionals/special-topics/hitech-act-enforcement-interim-final-rule/index.html.

Varker, T., Brand, R. M., Ward, J., Terhaag, S., & Phelps, A. (2019). Efficacy of synchronous telepsychology interventions for people with anxiety, depression, posttraumatic stress disorder, and adjustment disorder: A rapid evidence assessment. *Psychological Services, 16*(4), 621–635. https://doi.org/10.1037/ser0000239.

Waltman, S. H., Landry, J. M., Pujol, L. A., & Moore, B. A. (2019). Delivering evidence-based practices via telepsychology: Illustrative case series from military treatment facilities. *Professional Psychology: Research and Practice, 51*(3), 205–213. http://dx.doi.org/10.1037/pro0000275.

Weissman, R. S., Bauer, S., & Thomas, J. J. (2020). Access to evidence-based care for eating disorders during the COVID-19 crisis. *International Journal of Eating Disorders, 53*(5), 639–646. https://doi.org/10.1002/eat.23279.

Whitney, D. G., & Peterson, M. D. (2019). US national and state-level prevalence of mental health disorders and disparities of mental health care use in children. *JAMA Pediatrics, 173*(4), 389–391. https://doi.org/10.1001/jamapediatrics.2018.5399.

World Health Organization (WHO). (2019, November 28). Mental *d*isorders. Retrieved from www.who.int/news-room/fact-sheets/detail/mental-disorders.

Yuen, E. K., Herbert, J. D., Forman, E. M., Goetter, E. M., Juarascio, A. S., Rabin, S., … Bouchard, S. (2013). Acceptance based behavior therapy for social anxiety disorder through videoconferencing. *Journal of Anxiety Disorders, 27*(4), 389–397. https://doi.org/10.1016/j.janxdis.2013.03.002.

3   Guidebooks and Recommendations for Ethical and Legal Practice

In order for a provider to ensure the highest level of care, as well as protect their own practice, knowledge of both ethical and legal considerations of videoconferencing become vital. Both aspects present different, but often overlapping, components. While some ethical or legal considerations may seem obvious, others may not. Unfortunately, when it comes to telepsychology, the phrase "you don't know what you don't know" often becomes very pertinent, as specialized knowledge is required to fully understand the unique aspects of the processes. For example, consider a provider who transitioned from F2F to videoconferencing. They believe that they are great at providing assessments and therapy, and also very adept at using technology. Further, they have purchased top-of-the-line equipment, and created a new informed consent form to highlight the strengths and weaknesses of videoconferencing. They then begin providing services as they had in F2F interactions, with little modification. While the provider may have taken several steps to ensure proper practice, did they discuss the patient disclosing their location for each session to ensure that the care is being provided in states of the provider's license(s)? Have the provider and patient discussed billing should the services disconnect, resulting in sessions ending early? Does the provider have a clearly defined emergency plan with contact information for local emergency services in case a patient becomes volatile and abruptly logs off from the videoconferencing session? This example illustrates the importance of knowledge of the unique aspects of the videoconferencing processes, and a need to plan for such aspects to ensure an ethical, legal, and safe practice.

Guiding Organization Recommendations for Ethical Practice

Within the United States, ethical and legal guidance for videoconferencing practice can be viewed as evolving from one of the first documented formal guidebooks created in 2008 by the Ohio Psychological Association (OPA; Dielman et al., 2009). The guidebook reviewed the ethical and legal requirements for practice, informed consent and disclosures processes, secure communications and electronic transfer of patient information standards, access to and storage of communications protocols, fees and financial arrangements, and a set of interdisciplinary principles for professional practice. Recommendations have grown over time, with current guidance for telepsychology-related practices being available from several mental health-related organizations including the American Psychological Association (APA, 2013); the American Counseling Association (ACA, 2014); the collective of the National Association of Social Workers, the Association of Social Work Boards, the Council on Social Work Education, and the Clinical Social Work Association (NASW, ASWB, CSWE, & CSWA, 2017); the National Association of School Psychologists (NASP, 2017, 2020); the American Psychiatric Association (n.d.); and the American Telemedicine Association (ATA; Myers et al., 2017; Turvey et al., 2013; Yellowlees et al., 2010). Such documentation (Table 3.1) varies in content, ranging from full guidelines for general practice using technology (e.g., APA's *Guidelines for the Practice of Telepsychology* [2013]; NASW, ASWB, CSWE, & CSWA's *Standards for Technology in Social Work Practice* [2017]) to focused guidelines regarding specific aspects of videoconferencing work (e.g., ATA's *Practice Guidelines for Videoconferencing-Based Telemental Health*; *Practice Guidelines for Telemental Health with Children and Adolescents*).

Although each presents a differing focus (e.g., psychologist, social worker, counselor, psychiatrist), and level of detail, a review of each organization's documentation yields several broad themes to guide ethically and legally responsible practice: the need for competence and upholding of ethical standards, the clinical relationship, standards of care for the delivery of interventions, testing and assessment, informed consent, confidentiality, data security, disposal of data and hardware, logistics of practice, and

Table 3.1 Mental health applicable documentation

Organization	Document	Weblinks to documents
American Psychological Association (APA)	*Guidelines for the Practice of Telepsychology* (2013)	www.apa.org/practice/guidelines/telepsychology
National Association of Social Workers, Association of Social Work Boards, Council on Social Work Education, and the Clinical Social Work Association (NASW, ASWB, CSWE, & CSWA)	*NASW, ASWB, CSWE, & CSWA Standards for Technology in Social Work Practice* (2017)	www.socialworkers.org/LinkClick.aspx?fileticket=lcTcdsHUcng%3D&portalid=0
American Counseling Association (ACA)	*ACA Code of Ethics* (2014)	www.counseling.org/resources/aca-code-of-ethics.pdf

(*continued*)

Table 3.1 Cont.

Organization	Document	Weblinks to documents
National Association of School Psychologists (NASP)	*Guidance for Delivery of School Psychological Telehealth Services* (2017) *Telehealth: Virtual Service Delivery Updated Recommendations* (2020)	www.nasponline.org/assets/documents/Guidance_Telehealth_Virtual_Service_%20Delivery_Final%20(2).pdf www.nasponline.org/resources-and-publications/resources-and-podcasts/covid-19-resource-center/special-education-resources/telehealth-virtual-service-delivery-updated-recommendations
American Psychiatric Association	*Telepsychiatry Toolkit* (n.d.)	www.psychiatry.org/psychiatrists/practice/telepsychiatry/toolkit
American Academy of Child and Adolescent Psychiatry (AACAP)	*Practice Parameters for Telepsychiatry with Children and Adolescents* (Myers & Cain, 2008)	www.jaacap.org/article/S0890-8567(08)60154–9/pdf
American Telemedicine Association (ATA)	*Practice Guidelines for Video-Based Online Mental Health Services* (Turvey et al., 2013) *Practice Guidelines for Videoconferencing-Based Telemental Health* (Yellowlees et al., 2010) *Practice Guidelines for Telemental Health with Children and Adolescents* (Myers et al., 2017)	www.americantelemed.org/resources/practice-guidelines-for-video-based-online-mental-health-services-2/ www.americantelemed.org/resources/practice-guidelines-for-videoconferencing-based-telemental-health/ www.americantelemed.org/resources/practice-guidelines-for-telemental-health-with-children-and-adolescents/
Ohio Psychological Association (OPA)	*Telepsychology Guidelines* (Dielman et al., 2009)	https://telehealth.org/wpress/wp-content/uploads/2013/11/TelepsychologyGuidelinesApproved041208.pdf

Table 3.2 APA's *Guidelines for the Practice of Telepsychology Standards**

Guideline	Description
1	Psychologists who provide telepsychology services strive to take reasonable steps to ensure their competence with both the technologies used and the potential impact of the technologies on clients/patients, supervisees, or other professionals.
2	Psychologists make every effort to ensure that ethical and professional standards of care and practice are met at the outset and throughout the duration of the telepsychology services they provide.
3	Psychologists strive to obtain and document informed consent that specifically addresses the unique concerns related to the telepsychology services they provide. When doing so, psychologists are cognizant of the applicable laws and regulations, as well as organizational requirements that govern informed consent in this area.
4	Psychologists who provide telepsychology services make reasonable effort to protect and maintain the confidentiality of the data and information relating to their clients/patients and inform them of the potentially increased risks to loss of confidentiality inherent in the use of the telecommunication technologies, if any.
5	Psychologists who provide telepsychology services take reasonable steps to ensure that security measures are in place to protect data and information related to their clients/patients from unintended access or disclosure.
6	Psychologists who provide telepsychology services make reasonable efforts to dispose of data and information and the technologies used in a manner that facilitates protection from unauthorized access and accounts for safe and appropriate disposal.
7	Psychologists are encouraged to consider the unique issues that may arise with test instruments and assessment approaches designed for in-person implementation when providing telepsychology services.
8	Psychologists are encouraged to be familiar with and comply with all relevant laws and regulations when providing telepsychology services to clients/patients across jurisdictional and international borders.

Source: APA (2013).
Note: * Information is a summary.

legal considerations. Of note, despite a large portion of the documentation predominantly focusing on telehealth as broadly defined, the information is believed to be applicable to a range of technology-enhanced practices, including videoconferencing. Further, as indicated in the respective documents, the provided recommendations are meant to assist practice and professional behaviors, but are not necessarily absolute, exhaustive, or mandatory. Nevertheless, adherence is encouraged to foster the highest level of ethical and legal practice when utilizing videoconferencing. The following

Table 3.3 NASP's *Guidance for Delivery of School Psychological Telehealth Services* (and update)*

Recommendation

- Adhere to all professional ethics, standards, policies, and positions.
- Become knowledgeable of and follow licensure and certification requirements.
- Ensure access to high-quality technology.
- Obtain appropriate professional development to ensure competence in the delivery of telehealth services.
- Use validated assessment tools and methods.
- Maintain thorough documentation and legal/professional record-keeping practices.
- Ensure high degrees of privacy, confidentiality, informed consent, and security.
- Consider whether telehealth services are safe, effective, and appropriate.
- Obtain the appropriate licensure/certification – and, if needed, liability insurance – to cover telehealth services.
- Practitioners are cautioned to follow all HIPAA regulations, rather than just FERPA regulations. Ensuring secure technology is paramount, as is ensuring that appropriate informed consent is explained and obtained.
- Virtual service delivery requires close adherence to ethical standards. The same level of ethical and professional standards should apply to telehealth services as it does to in-person delivery of school psychological services.
- Practitioners of telehealth must be certified or licensed in both their state of residence and the state in which their client resides.

Source: NASP (2020, 2017).
Note: * Information is a summary.

is a summary of the broad themes pertinent to clinical practice. For a summary of specific organization's guiding principles, please see Table 3.2 (APA), Table 3.3 (NASP), Table 3.4 (NASW, ASWB, CSWE, & CSWA), Table 3.5 (ACA), and Table 3.6 (American Psychiatric Association). See Table 3.7 for a comparison of broad principles across the organizations' documentation.

The Need for Competence and Upholding of Ethical Standards

As a guide for all of the subsequent principles, each reviewed document highlights the need for anyone practicing with technology to take reasonable steps to ensure their competence with both the technologies themselves, and the potential impacts that the technology may hold for both the provider and the patient. To accomplish this, providers should seek research literature (Appendix F), books (Appendix F), formal training (e.g., graduate education, continuing education [CE] programming; Appendix G), consultation, and supervision. Specific foci of educational endeavors include, but are not limited to, the specific benefits of the technology-based approach; the limitations or risks associated with use of the technology; research on outcomes for specific diagnoses, ages, SES, cultures, languages,

Table 3.4 NASW, ASWB, CSWE, & CSWA Standards for Technology in Social
   Work Practice*

Section	Standards
1. Provision of information to the public	1.01 Ethics and values 1.02 Representation of self and accuracy of information
2. Designing and delivering services	2.01 Ethical use of technology to deliver social work services 2.02 Services requiring licensure or other forms of accreditation 2.03 Laws that govern provision of social work services 2.04 Informed consent: discussing the benefits and risk of providing electronic social work services 2.05 Assessing clients' relationships with technology 2.06 Competence: knowledge and skills required when using technology to provide services 2.07 Confidentiality and the use of technology 2.08 Electronic payments and claims 2.09 Maintaining professional boundaries 2.10 Social media policy 2.11 Use of personal technology for work purposes 2.12 Unplanned interruptions of electronic social work services 2.13 Responsibility in emergency circumstances 2.14 Electronic and online testimonials 2.15 Organizing and advocacy 2.16 Fundraising 2.17 Primary commitment to clients 2.18 Confidentiality 2.19 Appropriate boundaries 2.20 Addressing unique needs 2.21 Access to technology 2.22 Programmatic needs assessments and evaluations 2.23 Current knowledge and competence 2.24 Control of messages 2.25 Administration 2.26 Conducting online research 2.27 Social media policies
3. Gathering, managing, and storing information	3.01 Informed consent 3.02 Separation of personal and professional communications 3.03 Handling confidential information 3.04 Access to records within an organization 3.05 Breach of confidentiality 3.06 Credibility of information gathered electronically

(*continued*)

Table 3.4 Cont.

Section	Standards
	3.07 Sharing information with other parties
	3.08 Client access to own records
	3.09 Using search engines to locate information about clients
	3.10 Using search engines to locate information about professional colleagues
	3.11 Treating colleagues with respect
	3.12 Open-access information
	3.13 Accessing client records remotely
	3.14 Managing phased-out and outdated electronic devices
4. Social work education and supervision	4.01 Use of technology in social work education
	4.02 Training social workers about the use of technology in practice
	4.03 Continuing education
	4.04 Social media policies
	4.05 Evaluation
	4.06 Technological disruptions
	4.07 Distance education
	4.08 Support
	4.09 Maintenance of academic standards
	4.10 Educator–student boundaries
	4.11 Field instruction
	4.12 Social work supervision

Source: NASW et al. (2017).
Note: * Information is a summary.

*Table 3.5 ACA Code of Ethics**

Section	Standard
The counseling relationship	A.1 Client welfare
	A.2 Informed consent in the counseling relationship
	A.3 Clients served by others
	A.4 Avoiding harm and imposing values
	A.5 Prohibited noncounseling roles and relationships
	A.6 Managing and maintaining boundaries and professional relationships
	A.7 Roles and relationships at individual, group, institutional, and societal levels
	A.8 Multiple clients
	A.9 Group work
	A.10 Fees and business practices
	A.11 Termination and referral
	A.12 Abandonment and client neglect

Table 3.5 Cont.

Section	Standard
Confidentiality and privacy	B.1 Respecting client rights
	B.2 Exceptions
	B.3 Information shared with others
	B.4 Groups and families
	B.5 Clients lacking capacity to give informed consent
	B.6 Records and documentation
	B.7 Case consultation
Professional responsibility	C.1 Knowledge of and compliance with standards
	C.2 Professional competence
	C.3 Advertising and soliciting clients
	C.4 Professional qualifications
	C.5 Nondiscrimination
	C.6 Public responsibility
	C.7 Treatment modalities
	C.8 Responsibility to other professionals
Relationships with other professionals	D.1 Relationships with colleagues, employers, and employees
	D.2 Provision of consultation services
Evaluation, assessment, and interpretation	E.1 General
	E.2 Competence to use and interpret assessment instruments
	E.3 Informed consent in assessment
	E.4 Release of data to qualified personnel
	E.5 Diagnosis of mental disorders
	E.6 Instrument selection
	E.7 Conditions of assessment administration
	E.8 Multicultural issues/diversity in assessment
	E.9 Scoring and interpretation of assessment
	E.10 Assessment security
	E.11 Obsolete assessment and outdated results
	E.12 Assessment construction
	E.13 Forensic evaluation: evaluation for legal proceedings
Supervision, training, and teaching	F.1 Counselor supervision and client welfare
	F.2 Counselor supervision competence
	F.3 Supervisory relationship
	F.4 Supervisor responsibilities
	F.5 Student and supervisee responsibilities
	F.6 Counseling supervision evaluation, remediation, and endorsement
	F.7 Responsibilities of counselor educators
	F.8 Student welfare
	F.9 Evaluation and remediation
	F.10 Roles and relationships between counselor educators and students
	F.11 Multicultural/diversity competence in counselor education and training programs
Research and publication	G.1 Research responsibilities
	G.2 Rights of research participants

(continued)

Table 3.5 Cont.

Section	Standard
	G.3 Managing and maintaining boundaries
	G.4 Reporting results
	G.5 Publication and presentations
Distance counseling, technology, and social media	H.1 Knowledge and legal considerations
	H.2 Informed consent and security
	H.3 Client verification
	H.4 Distance counseling relationship
	H.5 Records and web maintenance
	H.6 Social media
Resolving ethical issues	I.1 Standards and the law
	I.2 Suspected violations
	I.3 Cooperation with ethics committees

Source: (ACA, 2014).
Note: * Information is a summary

Table 3.6 American Psychiatric Association's *Telepsychiatry Toolkit**

Section	Standard
History and background	History of telepsychiatry
	Advocacy issues
	Clinical outcomes
	Evidence base
	Feasibility and effectiveness
	Return on investment
Training	Adapting your practice, learning to do telemental health
	Credentialing process
	Media communication skills
	Style adaption
	Working with residents
Legal and reimbursement issues	Malpractice issues
	Medicaid reimbursement
	Private insurance reimbursement
	Ryan Haight Act
	State licensure
Technical considerations	Platform and software requirements
	Security issues
	Telepsychiatry and integration with other technologies
Practice and clinical issues	Child and adolescent telepsychiatry
	Clinical documentation
	Clinical and therapeutic modalities
	Geriatric telepsychiatry
	Individual models of care
	Inpatient telepsychiatry
	Patient safety and emergency management

Table 3.6 Cont.

Section	Standard
	Rural and remote practice settings Standard of care and state-based regulations Telepsychiatry practice guidelines Team-based integrated care Team-based models of care Use of telepsychiatry in cross-cultural settings Visual and nonverbal considerations

Source: American Psychiatric Association (n.d.).
Note: * Information is a summary.

Table 3.7 Overlap of primary ethical principles in mental health-focused guides related to telehealth practices*

Primary principle	APA	ACA	NASW, ASWB, CSWE, & CSWA	NASP	American Psychiatric Association
Ensure competence related to technologies and its impacts on care	X	X	X	X	X
Uphold ethical standards	X	X	X	X	X
Informed consenting practices	X	X	X	X	X
Administrative and documentation practices	X	X	X	X	X
Confidentiality and privacy practices	X	X	X	X	X
Data security	X	X	X	X	X
Data and hardware disposal	X	X	X	X	
Intervention considerations	X	X	X	X	X
Assessment considerations	X	X	X	X	X
Knowledge of relevant laws and standards including licensure standards	X	X	X	X	X
Ensure ongoing professional development	X	X	X	X	

(*continued*)

Table 3.7 Cont.

Primary principle	APA	ACA	NASW, ASWB, CSWE, & CSWA	NASP	American Psychiatric Association
Seek training, consultation, and supervision for new competencies	X	X	X	X	
Representation of provider's self to public		X	X		
Social media use		X	X	X	X
Conducting research		X			

Note: * Direct highlighting of topic in documentation.

and disability statuses; means of fostering a strong therapeutic alliance; differences in the application of technology-enhanced techniques as they compare to F2F care; and means of both preventing and addressing challenges, including emergency situations. Beyond these primary foci, part of this gained competency is also a recognition of one's boundaries of competence. Providers must reflect on their knowledge, realizing that rapid changes may quickly make their knowledge outdated. Further, while some providers may be adept at specific aspects of technology-based care, they may not be as knowledgeable on others.

The Clinical Relationship

The provider–patient relationship, also referred to as therapeutic alliance, has long been concluded as an essential component of positive clinical outcomes (Horvath & Luborsky, 1993; Lambert & Barley, 2001; Sharf et al., 2010). To ensure an appropriate relationship through technology, providers should take specific steps. First, they should explain potential differences between F2F and technology-based encounters, including the potential loss of certain nonverbal behaviors (e.g., leg bouncing that may be off camera). While summarizing these limitations, the provider should also take care to balance this information with indications that past research has demonstrated that the provider–patient relationship can effectively be built and maintained through technology mediums, including videoconferencing. Once services begin, the provider should take an active role in fostering the therapeutic alliance, including utilizing empathetic responding, ensuring active collaboration with the patient, and monitoring for rupture markers that may indicate that the patient is either experiencing difficulties, may not feel comfortable, or is disengaged with the processes. Such rupture markers may include overt or indirect expression of negative sentiment or hostility, disagreement about goals or tasks of the treatment, compliance issues, avoidance maneuvers (e.g., becoming oppositional or avoidant when discussing therapeutic processes), self-esteem-enhancing operations (e.g., self-justifying their own actions), and general nonresponsiveness to interventions (Safran et al., 1990; Safran et al., 2001). Finally, the provider should take care to consider, evaluate, and potentially remedy any dual relationships that may arise as a result of the use of the videoconferencing.

Standards of Care for the Delivery of Interventions

To uphold the highest standards of care, guiding organizations' documentation also indicates that providers should consider the unique issues that may arise with intervention approaches using technology. Applying their competence gained from education, providers must critically evaluate their practice in terms of how strategies must be adapted (e.g., how specific CBT techniques can be applied through videoconferencing), the limitations of this approach, and how these adaptations will compare to F2F methods. More directly related to the patient, the provider must also determine if such adaptations have been evaluated in the research for demographics similar to the patient, including age, sex, gender, diagnostic condition, and general history. Further, the provider should consider the role of cultural issues, as well as the potential influence of any comorbid cognitive, physical, or mental health-related challenges that may influence the treatment processes. Ultimately, such considerations can help ensure the appropriateness of the patient for the use of technology in their psychological care. In efforts to evaluate the technology-based strategies, the provider should implement targeted measurement. Such evaluation can not only focus on the clinical outcomes, but also technology-focused factors, such as the patient's comfort with the technology, as well as any changes in attitude related to either mental health or technology following usage. Critical evaluation is essential, as if gains are not made or sustained during treatment, the provider must consider whether issues are related to the technology use itself, or another factor, before considering a modification of their treatment plans.

Testing and Assessment

In supplement of interventions, the documentation calls for providers to consider the unique issues that may arise with testing instruments and assessment approaches when being conducted through technology-based means. This becomes especially pertinent when desired assessment measures were initially designed for F2F administration. As with standards of care for interventions, providers conducting assessments with the use of technology should evaluate the appropriateness of the patient for such procedures. This is especially important for patients with a recognized cognitive, physical, or mental health-related disability, in which the condition can interact with the technology to influence their score, limiting the provider's assessment of the patient's true ability (e.g., visual or hearing issues causing delayed performance and subsequent reduced scores). Points of evaluation related to the assessment materials should include the following: the assessment's procedures (e.g., does it requires manipulatives), if the assessments have been formally adapted for distance administration, if research has been completed on the distance administration, how to adapt the measures while maintaining the core principles of the test's administration, and the availability of normative data for distance administration. Further consideration should be given to the unique aspects of an online assessment, such as potential speed issues that could cause video or audio lags. Finally, when conducting a distance evaluation, consideration should be given to what the provider must see to ensure proper scoring of the assessment. For example, a provider may require multiple video devices to simultaneously observe the entire patient to monitor their general behavior, while also having a view focused on the patient's hands to evaluate their performance with manipulatives or written responses.

Informed Consent

Guiding organization documentation emphasizes the requirement of informed consent. Such consent should be conducted prior to the onset of the services, both verbally and in writing, and should be documented in the patient's medical record. In addition to standard informed consent protocols that are used for one's general F2F practice, telepsychology-specific informed consent processes should be implemented. The specialized informed consent is recommended to highlight several key aspects unique to the practice including, but not limited to, strength and limitations of the approach, differences between the technology-based method and F2F services, the research associated with the use of the desired technological modality, unique challenges with emergency situations and means of managing, methods of troubleshooting issues, and differences in billing for services. All information should be provided to the patient in language that is easily understandable for their developmental level and culture.

Confidentiality

Documentation also discusses that providers who use technology-based services make reasonable efforts to protect and maintain the confidentiality of the patient's protected health information (PHI). PHI may include patient names, addresses, phone numbers, email addresses, dates of birth, social security numbers, licenses, medical record number, digital identifiers, or biometric identifies (e.g., fingerprints, voice prints; Sivilli, 2018). Efforts to maintain confidentiality should include specific data security measures.

While a majority of the responsibility may fall to the provider, the patient should also be coached so that they can implement safeguards within their own settings.

Data Security

When using technology in clinical care, a range of potential data security issues can arise. As such, the provider should take extra caution and consideration of not only the methods being used to interact with the patient (e.g., email, videoconferencing, telephone), but the recorded data itself (e.g., notes in an EHR). Ultimately, the provider wants to restrict unintended access and disclosure of any PHI through physical safeguards (e.g., locks), technical safeguards (e.g., password systems), and administrative safeguards (e.g., trained staff).

Disposal of Data and Hardware

While basic storage of PHI is important, proper disposal of old data is also essential, as one cannot simply "shred" the digital information. Guiding documentation highlights the importance of making reasonable efforts to dispose of data, as well as the technological devices used to store the PHI in a way that prevents unauthorized access. This remains true whether the software (i.e., computer programs) or hardware (i.e., the computer or computer component such as a hard drive) will be reused or completely destroyed. Providers are encouraged to develop policies and procedures that adhere to any federal, state, or organization's regulations for proper destruction of the technology and data. These policies could include self-completed destruction, or the hiring of a third-party company specializing in the destruction of confidential information. Finally, the provider should document the steps they took for proper protection of the data.

Logistics of Practice

Documentation indicates that part of proper practice includes ensuring technology-specific logistics. More specifically, administrative policies should be created to detail methods of clinical documentation, methods of storing the documentation (e.g., paper files, EHR), policies for what is stored in the patient's chart (e.g., if email communication or texts from the patient are included), and safety measures to ensure data security and proper disposal. Further, administrative policies should include an indication of normal operating procedures. This detailing includes modification for technology-based services, such as office hours and methods of billing for services, including late arrivals, missed appointments, and how to bill should either the provider or patient experience technical difficulties.

Table 3.8 Links to US governmental regulations

Children's Online Privacy Protection Rule (COPPA)	www.ftc.gov/enforcement/rules/rulemaking-regulatory-reform-proceedings/childrens-online-privacy-protection-rule
Family Educational Rights and Privacy Act (FERPA)	www2.ed.gov/policy/gen/guid/fpco/ferpa/index.html
Health Information Technology for Economic and Clinical Health Act (HITECH)	www.hhs.gov/hipaa/for-professionals/special-topics/hitech-act-enforcement-interim-final-rule/index.html
Health Insurance Portability and Accountability Act (HIPAA)	www.hhs.gov/hipaa/index.html

Legal Considerations

Finally, documentation indicates that beyond ethics, providers should become familiar with all relevant laws and regulations in their jurisdiction(s). This recommendation highlights how it is not enough for a provider to merely be aware of ethical practice, but must also be aware of relevant laws that may be country-wide, or state specific. These laws can apply to licensure, to informed consent, and to the reasons for breaking confidentiality. Further, the laws govern what to do should a data breach occur. As jurisdictions vary on regulations, the provider is encouraged to fully explore all relevant laws unique to their location and license. In addition to state laws, common American acts to be knowledgeable of include the Health Insurance Portability and Accountability Act (HIPAA), the Family Education Rights and Privacy Act (FERPA), the Children's Online Privacy Protection Act (COPPA), and the HITECH Act (Table 3.8).

Non-universally Agreed Principle: Ensuring Ongoing Professional Development

Although not indicated in all of the reviewed documentation, many emphasized the need for ongoing professional development. As changes are common to the ethics, legality, and implementation of telepsychological practices, it is important that providers remain up to date. In order to accomplish this, they can gain additional knowledge through the reading of peer-reviewed literature in respected journals (Appendix F), books (Appendix F), CE programming (Appendix G), or consultation and/or supervision with providers who are more adept at the telepsychological practices.

Summary Points

- Guiding documentation exists to assist providers in conducting an ethical, legal, and safe provision of telepsychological services.

- While each guiding document varies in focus and specificity, overlapping principles include: the need to ensure competence in all aspects of practice (e.g., intervention, assessment, administrative, technology); knowledge of ethical and legal standards; implementation of administrative and documentation practices, including informed consent processes; and confidentiality and data security protocols.

References

American Counseling Association (ACA). (2014). *ACA code of ethics.* Retrieved from www.counseling.org/docs/default-source/default-document-library/2014-code-of-ethics-finaladdress.pdf?sfvrsn=96b532c_2.

American Psychiatric Association Work Group on Telepsychiatry. (n.d.). *Telepsychiatry toolkit.* Retrieved from www.psychiatry.org/psychiatrists/practice/telepsychiatry/toolkit.

American Psychological Association (APA). (2013). *Guidelines for the practice of telepsychology.* Retrieved from www.apa.org/practice/guidelines/telepsychology.

Dielman, M., Drude, K., Ellenwood, A. E., Imar, T., Lichstein, M., Mills, M. B. A., … Thomas, K. C. (2009). *Telepsychology guidelines.* Columbus, OH: Ohio Psychological Association. Retrieved from https://cdn.ymaws.com/ohpsych.org/resource/resmgr/files/covid-19/OPATelepsychologyGuidelines-.pdf.

Horvath, A. O., & Luborsky, L. (1993). The role of the therapeutic alliance in psychotherapy. *Journal of Consulting and Clinical Psychology, 61*(4), 561–573. https://doi.org/10.1037/0022-006X.61.4.561.

Lambert, M. J., & Barley, D. E. (2001). Research summary on the therapeutic relationship and psychotherapy outcome. *Psychotherapy: Theory, Research, Practice, Training, 38*(4), 357–361. https://doi.org/10.1037/0033-3204.38.4.357.

Myers, K., & Cain, S. (2008). Practice parameter for telepsychiatry with children and adolescents. *Journal of the American Academy of Child & Adolescent Psychiatry, 47*(12), 1468–1483. https://doi.org/10.1097/CHI.0b013e31818b4e13.

Myers, K., Nelson, E. -L., Rabinowitz, T., Hilty, D., Baker, D., Barnwell, S. S., … Bernard, J. (2017). American Telemedicine Association practice guidelines for telemental health with children and adolescents. *Telemedicine and e-Health, 23*(10), 779–804. https://doi.org/10.1089/tmj.2017.0177.

National Association of School Psychologists (NASP). (2017). *Guidance for delivery of school psychological telehealth services.* Retrieved from www.nasponline.org/assets/documents/Guidance_Telehealth_Virtual_Service_%20Delivery_Final%20(2).pdf.

National Association of School Psychologists (NASP). (2020). *Telehealth: Virtual service delivery updated recommendations.* Retrieved from www.nasponline.org/resources-and-publications/resources-and-podcasts/covid-19-resource-center/special-education-resources/telehealth-virtual-service-delivery-updated-recommendations.

National Association of Social Workers, Association of Social Work Boards, Council on Social Work Education, & Clinical Social Work Association (NASW, ASWB, CSWE, & CSWA) (2017). *NASW, ASWB, CSWE, & CSWA standards for technology in social work practice.* Retrieved from www.socialworkers.org/LinkClick.aspx?fileticket=lcTcdsHUcng%3D&portalid=0.

Safran, J. D., Crocker, P., McMain, S., & Murray, P. (1990). Therapeutic alliance rupture as a therapy event for empirical investigation. *Psychotherapy: Theory, Research, Practice, Training, 27*(2), 154–165. https://doi.org/10.1037/0033-3204.27.2.154.

Safran, J. D., Muran, J. C., Samstag, L. W., & Stevens, C. (2001). Repairing alliance ruptures. *Psychotherapy: Theory, Research, Practice, Training, 38*(4), 406–412. https://doi.org/10.1037/0033-3204.38.4.406.

Sharf, J., Primavera, L. H., & Diener, M. J. (2010). Dropout and therapeutic alliance: A meta-analysis of adult individual psychotherapy. *Psychotherapy: Theory, Research, Practice, Training, 47*(4), 637–645. https://doi.org/10.1037/a0021175.

Sivilli, F. (2018, May 19). Developing your basic HIPAA checklist. Retrieved from Telebehavioral Health Institute. https://telehealth.org/blog/basic-hipaa-checklist/.

Turvey, C., Coleman, M., Dennison, O., Drude, K., Goldenson, M., Hirsch, P., … Bernard, J. (2013). ATA practice guidelines for video-based online mental health services. *Telemedicine and e-Health, 19*(9), 722–730. https://doi.org/10.1089/tmj.2013.9989.

Yellowlees, P., Shore, J., & Roberts, L. (2010). Practice guidelines for videoconferencing-based telemental health, October 2009. *Telemedicine and e-Health, 16*(10), 1074–1089. https://doi.org/10.1089/tmj.2010.0148.

4 Factors to Consider in Order to Ensure an Ethical and Legal Videoconferencing Practice

As outlined in Chapter 3, documentation from guiding organizations provides recommendations for ethical, legal, and safe telepsychological practice. Although the information is helpful in broadly guiding providers, each document varies in levels of detail regarding how to actually conform to the recommendations, especially related to videoconferencing. Unfortunately, as of July 2020 there are no universally accepted documents detailing best practices. To assist providers, the following is a consolidation of recommendations and literature from field experts and guiding organizations, designed to provide information for common ethical and legal considerations that are relevant to videoconferencing services. Topics discussed include licensing and jurisdiction, cross-state practice and interjurisdictional compacts, evaluating patient appropriateness, informed consent, safety planning, data security, and additional considerations for ensuring an ongoing ethical and legal practice.

Licensing and Jurisdiction

Within the United States, while federal regulations provide broad laws related to psychological practice (e.g., HIPAA), each state supplements these laws through the creation and enforcement of licensure requirements. While recognized as important for any provider, the idea of jurisdiction (i.e., the geographic area of which an authority, such as a court, extends; Lehman & Phelps, 2005; Martin, 2003) becomes increasingly complex when one considers both the unique aspects of videoconferencing and ongoing legislative changes (Muoio, 2017). For example, can a provider legally practice across state lines within the United States? If one does practice videoconferencing across state lines, which laws apply under which circumstances? What does one do if there are conflicting laws among differing states, especially if it is in relation to a duty to warn? Which state has jurisdiction if a provider sees a patient in State A, but the provider is located in State B? Ultimately, these questions aren't always easy to answer.

Although the guiding organization's documentation is clear in the suggestion for providers to adhere to legal regulations, the question becomes how does one become aware of all relevant laws? National laws and acts, such as HIPAA, FERPA, COPPA, and HITECH can be found on US governmental websites (Table 3.8). To clarify state-based laws and regulations, one of the best means is for providers to either call the state directly, or consult the corresponding state-based governmental website that details the licensure and practice stipulations. Beyond general practice guidelines, nearly all states have some form of documentation specifically related to the use of technology in psychological care, although the verbiage may vary and can include terms such as "telehealth," "telebehavioral," "telemedicine," and "telepsychology." As the information can become complex, organizations have created state-based resources to better understand the legal regulations (Table 4.1). While such resources can be viewed as helpful, they are not to replace a provider's direct reading of the legal requirements of their jurisdiction(s). Of note, while some states dictate that providers must read the laws and regulation themselves without any additional licensure-based assessment of the provider's actual understanding of such laws and regulations, some states have telepsychology considerations built into their licensure tests in efforts to ensure a provider's technology-based knowledge if they are practicing in that specific state (e.g., Ohio).

Table 4.1 Helpful resources to find state-specific telepractice regulations

Organization or website resource	Link
National Consortium of Telehealth Resource Center's State Analysis	www.telehealthresourcecenter.org
American Telemedicine Association's Policy Center	www.americantelemed.org
Epstein, Becker, and Green's *Telemental Health Laws*	www.ebglaw.com/ telemental-health-laws-app/

Cross-State Practice

Once one establishes the general laws and regulations that guide their practice, one of the biggest questions among videoconferencing providers is the notion of cross-state work. Can one legally practice across states? The short answer is yes, but there are many caveats to this answer. For those providers only seeking brief, short-term services (≤ 30 days) for a patient outside of the provider's state of license, most states within the United States have adopted a temporary cross-state practice protocol, with such information found by either calling the licensing board, or finding the information on their respective websites (Campbell & Norcross, 2018). Alternatively, for those providers who will be conducting services with patients on an ongoing basis (i.e., >30 days), with the exception of specific governmental organizations that are subject to their own cross-state regulations (e.g., Veteran's Affairs, Indian Health Services, Department of Defense; Luxton et al., 2016, chap. 3), best practice suggests one of two primary options: multiple licenses or joining an interjurisdictional compact.

Multiple Licenses

The first primary option for legal cross-state practice involves the provider becoming licensed in all states in which they provide services. This means that if they are physically living in Illinois, but are providing services to patients in Illinois, Ohio, Texas, and Florida, the safest means of ensuring cross-state practice is securing licenses to practice in Illinois, Ohio, Texas, and Florida. In becoming licensed, the provider learns about the laws and regulations of each specific state. This becomes especially important when one considers that each of the states may have different regulations related to mandated reporting, emergency situations (e.g., involuntarily hospitalization), and red flag laws (i.e., a court can temporarily remove firearms from an individual). While becoming licensed in each state of practice may be a safe strategy, this approach could become costly both financially and in terms of time.

Interjurisdictional Compact

The second primary option for legal cross-state practice involves the provider becoming enrolled in a compact. To put it simply, a compact is a legal agreement between states that sign the compact into law. Any provider who is accepted as a member of the compact is under the compact's rules. Thus, a provider of the compact can practice across all states that are legally part of the compact without having to get individual licenses for each of the states. While some mental health organizations have introduced legislation (e.g., ACA Interstate Compact created by the National Center for Interstate Compacts and the Council of State Governments; Meyers, 2020), to date, one of the only fully implemented mental health-focused compacts uniquely applies to psychologists. The Psychological Interjurisdictional Compact, or PSYPACT (www.psypact.org/), was spearheaded by the Association of State and Provincial Psychology Boards (ASPPB), and formally introduced in February 2015. PSYPACT required seven states to enter the pact into law before it could be considered operational. As of its launch in July 2020, 15 states have enacted PSYPACT (i.e., Arizona, Colorado, Delaware, Georgia, Illinois, Missouri, Nebraska, New Hampshire, Nevada, Oklahoma, Texas Utah, Pennsylvania, Virginia, North Carolina), with 13 more locations having introduced legislation (i.e., Alabama, District of Columbia, Hawaii, Iowa, Kentucky, Michigan, Minnesota, New Jersey, Ohio, Rhode Island, Tennessee, Washington, West Virginia). Updates of legislative changes can be found at the PSYPACT website (https://psypact.org/page/psypactmap). PSYPACT created a means of cross-state practice through an Authority to Practice Interjurisdictional Telepsychology (APIT), which requires an active ASPPB E.Passport (ASPPB, 2016). To facilitate provider mobility, the PSYPACT states communicate and exchange information related to verification of licenses, necessary demographic information, and details of any disciplinary actions taken against the provider.

E. Passport

Per related ASPPB and PSYPACT documentation (ASPPB, 2020), to be eligible for an E.Passport, a provider must have an active license based on a doctoral degree in at least one PSYPACT state, with no disciplinary action listed against their license. Their degree must be from an APA or Canadian Psychological Association (CPA) accredited program, designated as a psychology program by the ASPPB/National Register Joint Designation Committee at the time of conferral, or deemed to be equivalent. The provider must have also successfully passed the Examination for Professional Practice in Psychology (EPPP). Finally, the program will require annual renewal with at least three hours of CE relevant to the use of technology in psychological practice. Assuming maintenance of qualification, the E.Passport is considered unlimited in time. Of important note, the provider will be subject to the scope of practice of the receiving state (i.e., originating site), which is the PSYPACT participating state where the patient is physically located when the services are delivered.

The Identification of Minimal Contact

Whether securing multiple licenses or joining a compact, knowledge of state regulations for cross-state work is important for two primary reasons. First, and most obvious, if a provider does not follow the regulations (e.g., licensing), they may be practicing illegally. Second, and equally as important, regardless of the license type, a provider may still be held liable in both the state that they are physically in (i.e., distant site), and the state of the patient (i.e., originating site) should an issue occur. For example, some have documented that attorney generals for many states have claimed jurisdiction even if the provider is from outside of the state (Koocher & Morray, 2000). Jurisdiction claims can be based on what some have termed "minimal contact." More specifically, a court may apply jurisdiction over a defendant who has no physical presence in a state as long as the defendant has engaged in purposeful actions in the state (Gupta & Sao, 2011; Kramer et al., 2013). Some have argued that videoconferencing providers who remotely diagnose and/or treat patients from another state are in fact establishing a minimal contact for the purposes of jurisdiction (Gupta & Sao, 2011).

Evaluating Patient Appropriateness

As providers aim to deliver the highest level of care, ensuring that the patient can benefit from videoconferencing services, while protecting their safety and privacy, is of critical importance (ATA, 2003). Unfortunately, not all patients will demonstrate qualities that make them good candidates. It is suggested that providers strive to have at least one initial F2F visit with the patient before transitioning to videoconferencing in order to evaluate their appropriateness for the technology-based services through both observations and information gathering (i.e., some patient factors may not be readily evident through alternative means). While having an initial F2F session is preferred, it may not always be possible, especially for those patients who live far distances from the provider, or lack either transportation or mobility. Regardless of whether it occurs F2F or through another means (e.g., telephone), providers should gather specific information regarding patient appropriateness before beginning videoconferencing services. Such information can be grouped into five primary categories: past clinical experiences of the patient, diagnostic considerations, technical considerations, setting considerations, and logistical considerations (Table 4.2; Lustgarten & Elhai, 2018; Luxton et al., 2016, chap. 3; Shore & Lu, 2015). While categories are not mutually exclusive, and some overlap of content exists, providers are recommended to evaluate all categories rather than focusing on just the clinical presentation or technological abilities of the patient. Although an appropriateness evaluation will take some additional time, this assessment can contribute to a successful outcome, as well as a happy patient, which could influence future referrals.

Table 4.2 Key factors to consider when evaluating a patient's appropriateness for videoconferencing

Factor	Description
Past clinical experiences	• General feelings towards mental health? • Has used technology in clinical care before? • If received F2F or online services, how did they like them?
Clinical	• Cognitive or sensory deficits? • Safety concerns (suicidal or homicidal ideation, firearms)? • Substance use/abuse? • High-risk diagnosis? • Clinical-related stability or volatility?
Technical	• Attitudes towards technology? • Have reasonable technology in their home? • Comfort with using technology? • Required and/or available technical aids (e.g., headsets)?
Setting	• Easily accessible? • Quiet? • Private? • Comfortable? • Well lit?
Logistical	• Barriers to care (e.g., financial, transportation, disability)? • Available patient support system?

Past Clinical Experiences of the Patient

As an initial step in determining a patient's appropriateness for videoconferencing, the provider should evaluate the patient's past clinical experiences and corresponding attitudes, both related to general psychological care, and if technology (e.g., videoconferencing, email) was integrated into any of this past work. To assess for attitudes towards psychology, the provider may start by questioning the patient's general feelings towards mental health, both broadly and more specifically related to either assessment or intervention. Further, the provider can question if the patient had ever received prior psychological services, and if they did, how they liked it. In supplement of this, the provider can ask how compliant the patient was with any recommendations from the past services. Such questions can help clarify not only feelings, but also the patient's past and current levels of motivation to engage in the treatment processes. Similarly, the provider can question if the patient has ever had technology integrated as part of prior psychological or medical care. If they had, what type of technology was used, when was it used, what was it for, how did the patient like it, what did they dislike about it, did the patient recognize any major issues that could have been addressed to improve the processes, and would they engage in similar services again? The provider can then directly ask if the patient would be interested in integrating videoconferencing into the current psychological care. Combining information can create a clearer picture of whether the patient is an appropriate candidate for the videoconferencing services. For example, if the patient is demonstrating reservations or resistance to the idea of general psychological services, beginning care with the additional complexities of videoconferencing may not be optimal if F2F alternatives are available and viable. Similarly, if the patient holds negative views of technology's integration with the psychological processes as based upon past usage, and their opinion do not change through a discussion of the positive outcomes from the research, the use of videoconferencing may not be the best approach for that specific patient at that point in time. Alternatively, some patients may view the technology medium as a benefit and a means of fostering comfort with the psychological processes. As these patients will not be in a physical room with a provider, they may enjoy the potential disinhibition that comes from the videoconferencing. Such an approach may be especially helpful for those who are willing to participate via videoconferencing, but hold a stigma related to psychological care and are thus not motivated to attend F2F services. For these individuals, providing a safe environment that is not the provider's office can be a means to begin treatment and foster both increased comfort and reduced misconceptions about the therapeutic processes (Collie, 2004; Suler, 2004).

Diagnostic Considerations

Supplementing past clinical experiences, diagnostic considerations must be assessed. These considerations can relate to both mental health and medical factors. First and foremost, the provider should evaluate if the patient is presenting with serious issues that would preclude general out-patient services, requiring a higher level of care. Simply put, if the patient is not suitable for F2F outpatient work, adding the complexity of videocon-ferencing is likely not a good idea. Such concerns may include if they are acutely violent, suicidal, or homicidal. Additional concerns that may create pause for general outpatient services include active psychosis including hallucinations or delusions (i.e., requiring pharmacological stabilization prior to therapy processes being implemented), or if they are actively util-izing substances that put them at risk for safety concerns or withdrawal-related medical complications.

Assuming the patient is suitable for general outpatient services, the provider should then consider the research related to the patient's specific mental health condition(s) that they will be required to assess or treat. Has the research demonstrated positive outcomes of an assessment or treatment related to the patient's presenting concerns? If it has, under what circumstances was it tested (e.g., was it of a population age and demo-graphic similar to the patient), and what were the outcomes? If the patient would be a general candidate for outpatient services, and the research supports the use of videoconferencing for their specific demographics and concerns, then the provider has a strong rationale for using the technology.

Compounding the mental health-focused concerns are physical consid-erations of the patient that may hinder effective videoconferencing. For some, disabilities can create auditory or visual impairments. While there are means to overcome many issues, methods of addressing the challenges (e.g., headphones for hearing impairments, gaining access to hearing aids, specific glasses or monitors for visual challenges, purchasing a larger and clearer computer monitor for visual clarity) may not be equally possible for all patients given their location and financial situation. If a physical disability can have a significant impact on the therapeutic processes, and modifications cannot be made, videoconferencing is likely not the best means of reaching the patient if other services are possible.

Finally, the provider must evaluate the patient for any cognitive issues that can create a range of additional videoconferencing-related challenges. First, informed consent may become an issue if the individual's cogni-tive abilities create difficulty for their understanding of the benefits and risks of a videoconferencing process. Second, one's cognitive abilities may create challenges for the logistics of setting up and implementing the videoconferencing technology, even with provider coaching. This is espe-cially pertinent for problem-solving of the technology as challenges arise, as issues with connectivity, the Internet, and the video camera itself are likely to occur and require remedy. Unfortunately, if such issues cannot be reasonably addressed, it could affect both the therapeutic relationship, as well as the outcomes for the treatment. As such, if a patient has mild cognitive issues, but generally understands the processes, is able to pro-vide informed consent, and can problem-solve as the need arises, they are likely appropriate candidates for the videoconferencing. Alternatively, if they demonstrate comprehension issues and problem-solving challenges, potentially evidenced by a history of general issues with daily living, the videoconferencing technology may become a detriment to the patient's care. However, even if cognitive issues present as impairing, videoconferencing may still be viable if others (e.g., family members, guardian, nurse) are available to assist the patient in the therapeutic and technical processes.

Technical Considerations

To build upon past and diagnostic factors that can influence videoconferencing, providers should directly evaluate the availability of appropriate technology, as well as the patient's technological knowledge. If the provider or a provider's organization is not supplying the patient with the videoconferencing equipment (e.g., loaned to patient during care), it is important that the patient has appropriate technology readily available within either their home or other location where they will be receiving the services. As further detailed in later chapters, reasonable technology includes a functional and secure computer system, a high-definition video and audio system, and high-speed internet. If the patient does not have access to such technology, the provider can evaluate what is available in order to determine if it is "good enough" to effectively conduct the videoconferencing services.

In addition to mere access to technology, what is the patient's general comfort with the use of technology in their daily lives? Are there cultural or financial factors influencing their decisions? What is their comfort specifically related to videoconferencing? Does the patient understand how it works and how to problem-solve the hardware or software if needed? If not, is the provider's initial coaching on technological set up and promise of helping problem-solve if issues arise enough to build a level of comfort for the patient to utilize the videoconferencing for their care? Finally, and related to a patient's condition, does the use of technology itself create secondary issues? For example, is the technology causing additional stress for a patient with OCD (e.g., obsessive thoughts of if the system were to "crash" creating difficulties for focusing during sessions) or psychosis (e.g., paranoia about computer security issues). While such issues may be part of the assessment or intervention itself, the provider should consider if this lack of comfort will severely impair the processes, or if the use of technology will exacerbate difficulties and complicate treatment for those with more severe pathology (Hidy et al., 2013).

Setting Considerations

Just as a patient has clinical and technical considerations that make them better or worse candidates for videoconferencing, so too does the setting. The provider should inquire about where a patient is able to receive the videoconferencing services. As further detailed in Chapter 12, the setting should be easily accessible, quiet, comfortable (e.g., increased size for more people), well lit, and most importantly, private. This notion of privacy not only includes the patient's ability to sit in a room without interruption from either noise (e.g., loud television in another room) or others (e.g., family members, friends, siblings), but ideally a setting where the sessions cannot be easily heard through a wall or observed through a window. As such, a home, office, or local clinic are likely desirable settings, while sitting in a coffee shop or other public location would not be appropriate. Unfortunately, noise or a lack of privacy cannot only create distractions, but may also lead to a patient feeling less safe in the therapeutic processes (whether for individual therapy or group sessions involving others), prompting them to become less engaged and sharing of information. Ultimately, if a patient does not have an appropriate setting for the videoconferencing sessions, the provider should consider whether the services are the best option if other possibilities are available.

Logistical Considerations

As some of the most frequently cited reasons for utilizing videoconferencing relate to a patient's transportation issues, or limited access to providers in their areas, such considerations should also be evaluated. If the patient cannot physically get to a provider's office, whether it be due to transportation issues, a provider being too far from their home, financial reasons, or psychological or medical disability related, then videoconferencing may present a viable alternative.

An additional logistical consideration relates to the patient's level of support from others. Support could be from spouses, family, or community members. Supportive tasks throughout a psychological treatment can include assisting the patient with general day-to-day coping, or helping calm and stabilize them in more severe situations. This is especially important for higher-risk patients, or for crises that may arise. Unfortunately, not all patients have a strong support system. As such, the provider must consider whether videoconferencing is best for a higher-risk patient if alternative services are available, even if they are willing to reconsider and reevaluate the use of videoconferencing in the future once the patient becomes more stable.

Structured Guide for the Assessment of Suitability for Home-Based Telemental Health (ASH-25)

As there are numerous aspects of a patient to assess when it comes to videoconferencing appropriateness, although some providers may create their own lists of questions, some providers may desire a more structured protocol. While limited works are available specifically for telepsychological care, one unique tool is the ASH-25 (Shore & Lu, 2015; Figure 4.1). The ASH-25 is a 25-item provider-completed questionnaire encompassing both objective and subjective clinical observations to evaluate the patient

ASH-25, A Structured Guide for the Assessment of Suitability for Home-Based Telemental Health

Each question should be viewed as a variable in determining the level of risk the patient may pose in terms of a psychiatric and/or medical emergency.

EXAMINER: _____   Date: _____

NAME: _____

There are several variables that comprise a goodness of fit between a patient seeking care and the treating clinician. Please fill out according to your direct knowledge, either by way of medical records/review, interview with patient, their previous and/or current and/or former providers.

Background

1) REFERRAL SOURCE: primary care ( ) mental health clinic ( ) examiner ( )
2) AGE _____
3) DISABILITY _____% _____
4) Miles to nearest clinic _____
5) Miles to nearest medical center _____
6) Would the patient have received your services if otherwise not offered in the home or nonclinical setting? YES ( ) NO ( )
7) Does the patient have access to additional resources for treatment in their community? YES ( ) NO ( )
8) If yes to #7, please list: _____
9) What is the patient's primary reason for seeking services in the home or nonclinical setting? _____
10) In the patient's own words, describe any perceived stigma associated with receiving healthcare.

_____

Figure 4.1 Structured Guide for the Assessment of Suitability for Home-Based Telemental Health (ASH-25).

Note: BDI = Beck's Depression Inventory; MST = multisystemic therapy; PCL = PTSD Checklist; PSP = psychological support for personality; PTSD = post-traumatic stress disorder; tx hx = treatment history; VA = Veterans Affairs.

Source: Adapted from Shore and Lu (2015). Used with permission.

Please circle the response that best represents your interpretation and objective information pertaining to each variable. Please note: active substance abuse/dependence, active suicidal ideation with intent, and untreated thought disorders are exclusion factors.

Factor I: Mental Health

1. PRIMARY MENTAL HEALTH DIAGNOSIS: _____

0 Thought disorder (untreated or difficult to manage). Substance use/abuse dependence (current, recent), PTSD (chronic, MST, untreated/or minimal tx hx).

1 Axis II disorder and/or traits; PTSD (moderate); substance use dependence (nonalcohol); bipolar disorder (untreated, not well treated); serious mental illness (untreated, not well treated).

2 PTSD (not chronic); substance use disorders (in remission).

3 Depressive disorders/anxiety disorders.

If substance use present, please describe type, frequency, etc.:

_____

2. PSYCHIATRIC HOSPITALIZATIONS

0 Hospitalizations within last 30 days.

1 Hospitalizations 31 days to previous 6 months.

2 Remote history of hospitalization.

3 No history.

3. MOTIVIATION FOR MENTAL HEALTH TREATMENT (CURRENT)

0 Ambivalent

1 Pre-contemplative.

2 Contemplative (provider recommended treatment and home-based program).

3 Action (veteran requested treatment).

4 Maintenance (transfer from current mental health provider).

Figure 4.1 Continued

4. PREVIOUS MENTAL HEALTH TREATMENT COMPLIANCE

0 Multiple cancellations/no-shows.

1 Variable no-shows/cancellations (difficult to determine pattern).

2 Relatively compliant (pattern consistent with good compliance, but occasional).

3 Compliant.

5. PREVIOUS MENTAL HEALTH TREATMENT SUCCESS/FAILURE

0 Multiple drop-outs of time-limited treatments.

1 Majority of failures/incomplete treatments.

2 Variable successes/failures to complete.

3 Majority of successes/completion of treatments.

6. PATIENT'S SUBJECTIVE PERSPECTIVE ON STIGMA

0 Perceived stigmas correlated with no interest in receiving mental health treatment.

1 Perceived stigma, but veteran would only receive mental health treatment in home.

2 Perceived stigma, but veteran comfortable with receiving mental health treatment in VA facility.

3 No perceived stigma.

7. MOOD INVENTORY SCORES: MOST RECENT PCL/DATE: _____ MOST RECENT BDI/DATE: _____

0 BDI, PCL, or other measures significantly elevated within last 30 days.

1 BDI, PCL, or other measures significantly elevated 31 days to 6 months.

2 BDI, PCL, or other measures mild to moderately elevated within last 30 days.

3 BDI, PCL, or other measures within normal range.

8. COGNITIVE FUNCTIONING

0 Significant deficits.

1 Moderate deficits.

2 Mild deficits.

3 Within normal range.

Figure 4.1 Continued

9. SUICIDE HISTORY

0 Recent active ideation/attempt. High risk: YES/NO.

1 Remote ideation/attempt.

2 Passive ideation/low lethality.

3 Denies ideation (remote).

4 Denies ideation (current, recent).

10. DISRUPTIVE BEHAVIOR HISTORY (aggressive behavior, drug-seeking behavior, or behaviors interfering with the receipt or delivery of healthcare)

0 Recent history (within 60 days). Legal involved.

1 Recent history (within 61 days to a year). No legal.

2 Remote history (over a year). Legal involved.

3 No history.

11. NEW MENTAL HEALTH DIAGNOSIS (within 60 days):

_____

12. INITIAL MENTAL HEALTH TREATMENT PLAN:

_____

Factor II: Medical

13. CURRENT MEDICAL STATUS

0 Medically compromised, requires assistance with daily functioning.

1 Medically compromised, requires partial assistance with daily functioning.

2 Medical conditions well treated/managed; patient independent.

3 Medically clear, no secondary interventions.

14. PREVIOUS MEDICATION COMPLIANCE

0 Multiple records of noncompliance.

Figure 4.1 Continued

1 Variable compliance (due to extraneous factors such as complicated medical).

2 Relatively compliant (pattern consistent with good compliance, but occasional miss).

3 Compliant.

15. MEDICAL COMPLICATIONS (within 60 days):

Factor III: Access to Care

16. BARRIERS TO CARE

0 Financial limitations (can't afford gasoline).

1 Without transportation, limited resources for childcare.

2 Geographic hardship (approximately 60+ miles to closest clinic, difficult travel terrain).

3 Physical limitations, chronic medical and/or psychiatric conditions.

4 Homebound.

17. COMFORT WITH PERSONAL COMPUTER/TECHNOLOGY

0 Doesn't feel comfortable.

1 Rarely uses computer/technology.

2 Some comfort level with computer/technology, but relies on others.

3 Checks email regularly, surfs the Internet, working knowledge of personal computer.

4 Sophisticated understanding of computer/technology; uses it daily and integrated into routine.

Factor IV: Systems

18. FAMILY

0 No family contact.

1 Family geographically diverse, not physically close.

2 Family located locally.

3 Lives with family.

Figure 4.1 Continued

19. SOCIAL NETWORK

0 Avoidant, isolates, unemployed.

1 No current relationship.

2 Some friends, passive relationships.

3 Friends, deeper/meaningful relationships.

4 Friends, wide network, active in community.

20. CURRENT LIVING SITUATION

0 Alone.

1 Roommate (nonrelationship, family member in negative standing).

2 Roommate (nonsexual relationship, family member in positive standing).

3 Significant other (relatively unstable)

4 Partnered, married (stable relationship).

21. STABILITY OF SYSTEM

0 Family and/or social network unreliable; fractured.

1 Individual family member and/or social network moderately reliable/stable.

2 Multiple family members and/or social network moderately reliable/stable.

3 Individual family members and/or social network reliable/stable.

4 Multiple family members and/or social network reliable/stable.

22. MILES TO EMERGENCY PERSONNEL (fire, paramedic, police, sheriff) _____ 0–1–2–3

23. PSP RELATIONSHIP STATUS

0 Acquaintance.

1 Neighbor (not regular social contact).

2 Friends/family (stable relationship).

3 Significant other (stable relationship).

24. PSP DISTANCE IN MILES/TIME TO PATIENT _____/_____ 0–1–2–3

Figure 4.1 Continued

25. PSP EXPERIENCE WITH CRISIS

0 No experience.

1 Some experience (nonlife-threatening).

2 Some experience (lift-threatening).

3 Numerous experiences (life-threatening).

EXAMINER COMMENTS:

_____

FINDINGS:

Total score: _____

Approved: _____

Approved (conditional): _____

      Conditions of approval: _____

Temporary denial: _____

Denial: _____

Date: _____

Figure 4.1 Continued

for nonclinic settings, such as their home. Patients are assessed across five primary domains: mental health, medical considerations, access to care, systems (e.g., family, community), and patient support system. While the ASH-25 is not normed, higher scores have been indicated to be suggestive of higher complexity of the patient.

Informed Consent

From an ethical and legal standpoint, given the unique nature, informed consent is one of the most vital considerations for the use of videoconferencing in patient care. Despite this importance, there are no recognized universal standards for what must be included in the informed consent process. Nevertheless, through a synthesis of works by guiding organizations, research, and field experts (e.g., APA, 2020; Jacobs, n.d.; Luxton et al., 2016, chap. 3; Murphy & Pomerantz, 2016), several specific recommendations and content areas arise.

Videoconferencing-Specific Informed Consent Factors

As novel methods are being added to treatment-as-usual approaches for a provider's practice, combined with the inherent changes in benefits, risks, and challenges that may occur from adding the technology, it is suggested that providers implement videoconferencing-specific informed consent processes. This means that providers should not rely on their traditional F2F informed consent forms and merely explain differences of the addition of technology to the patient. The videoconferencing-specific informed consent can be accomplished by either creating a new form that integrates information for both F2F and telepsychological encounters, or creating a telepsychology-specific supplemental form that is unique to the technology-based services. In either situation, it is important that the technology is highlighted above and beyond traditional practice. As technology-specific discussions can sometimes become complex, it is recommended that the provider create the informed consent forms at a readily understandable reading level, and ideally in the patient's native language (i.e., different translations of the informed consent forms). While there are few indications for what reading level is appropriate, in line with research requirements of numerous universities and medical centers (e.g., Johns Hopkins Medicine, 2016), government organizations (e.g., US Food & Drug Administration, 2014), and suggestions by researchers (e.g., Hochhauser, 2007; Tamariz et al., 2013), providers should try to not exceed a reading level of sixth to eighth grade, if possible. While different means are available to evaluate the reading level, one of the easiest is to

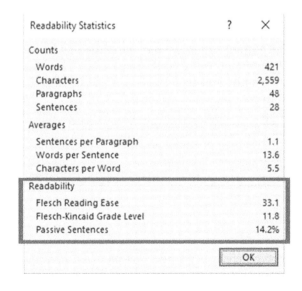

Figure 4.2 Sample Microsoft Word readability score.

enable "readability statistics" in Microsoft Word in the option settings. When a provider conducts a spelling and grammar check of the document, readability statistics will also be produced that lists the "Flesch-Kincaid Grade Level" (Figure 4.2).

Providing Both Verbal and Written Consent

As patients will present with different reading levels and attention to detail, it is suggested that providers supply the informed consent information both in writing and verbally. For those who prefer visual information, patients can read the details of the videoconferencing through the forms. Documents can then be signed either physically, or through a teleconsenting platform (e.g., DocuSign), with copies being placed into the patient's medical record, as well as provided to the patient. Information can also be provided verbally to supplement and clarify what is detailed in the forms. This method can help accommodate those who may experience attention-, reading-, or language-related challenges that may preclude them from fully grasping all information presented on the forms alone. Of particular importance, the provider should invite questions, feedback, concerns, or criticism, as addressing each prior to the onset of treatment can help calm the patient's nerves and foster the potential for improved outcomes. Further, this approach allows the patient to better understand the process and feel like more of a collaborator, which can foster their investment in the therapeutic processes (DeFife & Hilsenroth, 2011; Henry et al., 2017; Tryon & Winograd, 2011).

Content of the Informed Consent

As far as specific components to include in the informed consent, the literature, combined with helpful resources and checklists (Table 4.3), has highlighted several key content areas. Such areas relate to indications of general practices, strengths and limitations, general delivery factors, communication, troubleshooting, and administrative policies (Table 4.4; Luxton et al., 2016, chap. 3; Murphy & Pomerantz, 2016). Of note, not all discussed points may apply to all providers. Further, the level of specificity may be seen by some as excessive. As such, providers must tailor the information to their specific practices. The following is adapted for videoconferencing practice, but may also apply to other telepsychological methods (e.g., telephone).

Indication of General Practice

When indicating general practices, a provider should detail what types of videoconferencing services are and are not provided. This applies not only to specific ages and conditions treated, but also the therapy types offered

Table 4.3 Informed consent resources

Organization	Resource	Weblink
American Psychological Association	Informed consent checklist for telepsychological services	www.apa.org/practice/programs/dmhi/research-information/informed-consent-checklist
California Telehealth Resource Center	Sample forms and guidelines	www.caltrc.org/knowledge-center/best-practices/sample-forms/
National Association of Social Workers	Sample telemental health informed consent	www.socialworkers.org/LinkClick.aspx?fileticket=fN67-dWQReM%3D&portalid=0
National Association of Social Worker's Assurance Services	Sample telehealth informed consent	https://naswassurance.org/pdf/telehealth-informed-consent.pdf
Trust Parma	Sample informed consent form	https://parma.trustinsurance.com/Resources/Articles/sample-informed-consent-form
Trust Risk Management Services	Sample telehealth consent forms	www.trustrms.com/Resources/Articles/sample-telehealth-consent-forms
Upper Midwest Telehealth Resource Center	Sample informed consent for telemedicine services	www.umtrc.org/clientuploads/Resources/Sample%20Forms%20and%20Templates/Sample_Informed_Consent_for_Telemedicine_Services.pdf

(e.g., individual, group, family, couples), as well as assessments that one feels comfortable utilizing as based upon the research and available resources. Further, the information can outline if the provider is able to conduct more specialized videoconferencing services including forensic evaluations or custody work. If a provider is to utilize more than just videoconferencing services, they should be clear in what types are acceptable, such as emailing, texting, messaging programs, or telephone. Complementing this indication should be a discussion of which platforms a provider will or will not use. This information could include specific names of products, or specific criteria of what the provider approves of in such products, such as a certain level of security. As a provider can never be sure of future changes in such products, in lieu of being specific, one could merely indicate that telepsychological platforms are based upon the provider's judgment and are subject to change in order to account for cost increases or issues related to the platforms. Regardless of the types and setup, it is also suggested that the informed consent include a clause related to the fact that the patient agrees to receive the psychological services only in the agreed-upon states that the provider is able to supply legal services in (i.e., licensed in, states of an entered compact). This clause can detail that the patient agrees to disclose when they are either planning to be outside of the provider's licensed areas, or are already outside of the licensed jurisdiction before the services are delivered. Finally, the informed consent forms may indicate if the provider is supplying supervision to any trainees that may participate in the services of the patient.

Strengths and Limitations

To ensure that patients have appropriate knowledge of the videoconferencing practices in order to make an informed decision about their participation, an indication of both the strengths and limitations should be presented that aligns with contemporary literature. While one does not need to outline the research findings in detail, the informed consent should give an indication that telepsychology and videoconferencing services are still considered emerging fields with developing scientific literature. As such, there are gaps in knowledge. Nevertheless, with the rapid expansion of study of telepsychology over the past 20 years, researchers have suggested that there is currently enough literature to reasonably indicate that the videoconferencing can be effective for a wide range of conditions and ages, as long as it is conducted under specific circumstances and with considerations of noted limitations (Backhaus et al., 2012; Berryhill et al., 2019; Duncan et al., 2014; Turvey, 2018). Patients should be made aware that benefits may include, but are not limited to, the following: convenience, potentially improved access and less wait for general services, potentially improved access and less wait for specialized services, the ability of providers to reach patients where they are, economic benefits of a patient's reduced transportation-related expenses, reduced stress associated with transportation (e.g., traffic), and the potential for the patient to disclose more information through the research noted disinhibition effect (Bischoff et al., 2004; Feijt et al., 2018; Perle & Nierenberg, 2013). Contrastingly, patients should also be made aware that potential limitations may include, but are not limited to: the potential for interruptions during the session; the potential for people to listen in on the session, whether purposefully or accidentally; the potential for technology-related difficulties (e.g., video or audio issues, drops in connections); the potential for physical issues related to eyestrain from viewing the video display screen for extended periods of time; the potential reduction in the provider and patient's ability to see nonverbal cues that are more evident during F2F services; the potential for increased costs of securing proper equipment for the videoconferencing; the lack of a "cool-down" period (e.g., traveling home after session) following the end of the session that may occur during F2F services; the ongoing changes to ethical and legal standards; the need for additional research on the various aspects and implementation methods of the videoconferencing; and finally, the potential for someone to hack the technology and gain access to session content (Backhaus et al., 2012; Feijt et al., 2018; Perle et al., 2011).

General Delivery Factors

Supplementing the benefits and limitations, in order for a patient to have "informed" consent, they must be made aware of what aspects of the video-conferencing will be similar to F2F processes (e.g., therapeutic techniques), and which may differ (e.g., preventative emergency planning, sessions start with a video and audio check, collaborative role play may require more effort than in F2F interactions), as unique to the provider's practice. Building from the discussion of differences, technical factors should be highlighted as required for the delivery of the videoconferencing services. In doing so, the provider should indicate the minimum technical hardware and software specifications in readily understandable language. For example, a provider can indicate that the patient must download "_____" videocon-ferencing platform from "_____" weblink, while also indicating for this to run smoothly, the patient must have at least "_____" operating system (e.g., Windows version, Apple version). The provider can also specify which browsers are recommended if running the videoconferencing directly from the Internet (e.g., Google Chrome, Safari, Internet Explorer). There may also be a clause indicating that if the patient is unsure of specifications, they should consult the provider who can supply general guidance and help coach. As the use of technology allows for multiple means for a patient to contact a provider, it is also important to clarify what information will be included in the medical record to avoid misunderstandings. For example, a provider may use email or text communication as part of their videocon-ferencing treatment (i.e., between sessions). While many providers will con-sider this information part of the patient's care, some patients may not fully realize that all of these communications can be documented. Ultimately, through a review of combined noted information, it is possible that a patient may simply not feel comfortable using the videoconferencing. For such situ-ations, alternatives must be detailed, whether they be for F2F services with the same provider, or a referral to another healthcare provider. Finally, it is the provider's responsibility to ensure the patient's safety and care. As such, they may wish to include a clause in the informed consent forms indi-cating that they have the right to limit the use of videoconferencing (or other telepsychology) and provide alternative options should they believe that such services are no longer beneficial to the patient (i.e., gains not being achieved or sustained), if the services are believed to be more detrimental than helpful, or if there is a safety concern associated with ongoing use of videoconferencing as a result of the patient's unique situation.

Communication

Informed consent regarding communication should be viewed as especially important in order to maintain appropriate boundaries and professionalism (Drum & Littleton, 2014; Huggins, 2016; Luxton et al., 2016, chap. 3). As boundaries are key to effective practice, the patient must understand that merely because the provider is more readily available via telepsychology modalities (e.g., videoconferencing, telephone, email, messaging), does not necessarily mean that the provider is available to them at any moment. For example, while the videoconferencing sessions can be completed outside of the provider's usual business hours since they can conduct it from their home, does not mean that the provider should or will engage in such activities. Due to this, establishing hours of work, and the average turnaround time for communications can help clarify practices for the patient. In doing so, the provider may indicate that they will return all communications within a set amount of time as long as they are not on vacation, ill, or managing a crisis situation of another patient. Further, the provider can indicate that they may only answer messages within normal business hours for their practice. However, to plan for crises, the provider should outline how the patient can contact them outside of normal business hours, as well as what methods of communication may be appropriate or inappropriate for any correspondences. For example, the provider should include stipulations in the informed consent forms regarding what types of information is appropriate for email or texting, if those services are allowed for between-session communication. The forms can clearly indicate that if a patient is experiencing serious issues that do not warrant higher-level care through an emergency department (e.g., benign suicidal or homicidal ideation), a telephone or video call is necessary, with delayed messaging (e.g., email, texting) being inappropriate due to the need for a more immediate response. While some may merely choose to restrict usage of asynchronous modalities altogether, for those providers that allow use, the patient should be made aware that such messages are often not immediate and may either be delayed or not sent at all. As such, in addition to the provider's indication of a standard response time for communications, they should include a statement that if a patient does not hear back by a certain time, they are suggested to follow-up with a second message, potentially through a synchronous method.

Troubleshooting

Even with the best of planning, providers and patients are likely to encounter technological issues that require troubleshooting. As such, part of the informed consent process should describe what to do if the initially selected videoconferencing platform or equipment become unreliable. For instance, common issues often relate to a provider's or patient's video or audio quality, or one having a poor videoconferencing connection. To remedy such issues, the patient and provider can first attempt to reconnect and/or lower video or audio settings. In order for the provider to communicate how to do this during the videoconferencing disruption, the patient agrees to have their phone and email readily available during all sessions. Should the issues persist, the patient agrees to try a secondary provider-suggested videoconferencing platform. Should that not work, the patient agrees to utilize telephone-based services for that specific session, unless a designated amount of time has passed requiring the patient to merely reschedule due to remaining time limitations. While troubleshooting steps and policies are ultimately the provider's decision, such discussions can potentially be negotiated with the patient so they feel like collaborators in their own care. To ensure that the patient does not forget the steps, a copy of the forms can be provided that not only outlines the primary means of problem-solving general issues, but also includes a list of the proposed alternatives that are acceptable in case of complete equipment failure, or other concern limiting the agreed-upon services (e.g., accident, catastrophe, natural disaster).

Administrative

Although particular attention should be paid to the direct care aspects of one's practice, informed consent should also include a focus on administrative policies. These policies can cover a range of functions, but are especially pertinent to attendance expectations and associated billing practices. As research has clarified that a patient's attendance is an essential component for positive outcomes (Oldham et al., 2012; Reardon et al., 2002), providers should document what is an appropriate timeframe for a cancellation of a videoconferencing appointment. Further, they should detail what steps they will take (e.g., call via telephone, email, no action) and how long they will wait before considering the patient a "no-show." This indication can also suggest that the provider will check every set number of minutes to see if the patient "arrived." In doing so, the provider is indicating that they may be away from the videoconferencing system until the designated times to allow for ongoing productivity related to other matters.

Complementing the scheduling information is a detailing of how the provider will bill for the videoconferencing services. Is the provider paneled with the patient's insurance company? If not, will the videoconferencing sessions be billed with a similar fee schedule as F2F services, or are there differences in costs? As part of this billing process, the provider should also detail charges for cancellations, missed appointments, or no-charge situations. While a general statement indicating that videoconferencing billing will align with F2F practices may be sufficient, some providers may desire more flexibility. For example, does a provider bill the full session, or potentially a partial fee, if the patient's internet connection and phone service verifiably go down? Some may see this as outside of the patient's control and suggest that this should be a reduced or no-charge situation. Alternatively, some may see this as a "billable booked hour" in which the provider should get paid, as if they do not, it could be problematic for their finances or productivity ratings (e.g., relative value units).

Safety Planning

As detailed throughout the informed consent process, crises and emergency situations may arise requiring a provider's swift response, potentially

Table 4.4 Summary of recommended videoconferencing-specific informed consent
content areas

Factor	Specific components
Indication of general practice	• Detailing of the types of diagnoses treated and not treated • Detailing of the ages treated and not treated • Detailing of the types of therapy services provided and not provided • Detailing of the types of assessments provided and not provided • Detailing of the types of other telepsychological services provided or not provided • Detailing of what platforms or products are acceptable and not acceptable for services • Indication that the patient agrees to only receive services within agreed upon locations in which the provider is licensed • Indication that the patient agrees to disclose if they are or will be outside of the provider's licensed jurisdiction prior to receiving services • Indication of trainee involvement, if applicable
Strengths and limitations	• Indication that videoconferencing is an emerging scientific literature with limitations • Discussion of the potential benefits of the use of videoconferencing, including convenience, potentially improved access and less wait for general services, potentially improved access and less wait for specialized services, the ability of providers to reach patients where they are, economic benefits of a patient's reduced transportation-related expenses, reduced stress associated with transportation (e.g., traffic), and the potential for the patient to disclose more information through the research noted disinhibition effect • Discussion of the potential limitations of the use of videoconferencing, including the potential for interruptions during session, the potential for people to listen in on the session whether purposefully or accidentally, the potential for technology-related difficulties (e.g., video or audio issues, drops in connections), the potential for physical issues related to eyestrain from viewing the video screen for extended periods of time, the potential reduction in the provider and patient's ability to see nonverbal cues that are more evident during F2F services, the potential for increased costs of securing proper equipment for the videoconferencing, the lack of a "cool-down" period (e.g., traveling home after session) following the end of the session that may occur during F2F services, the ongoing changes to ethical and legal standards, the need for additional research on the various aspects and implementation methods of the videoconferencing, and the potential for someone to hack the technology and gain access to session content

Table 4.4 Cont.

Factor	Specific components
General delivery factors	• Description of how videoconferencing differs from F2F • Indication of the minimum technical specifications for hardware, software, and network • Indication of what will and will not go into medical record • Provisions for crises • Inclusion of a clause of alternatives if videoconferencing is deemed inappropriate
Communication	• Detailing of boundaries for interactions (i.e., hours of work, etc.) • Detailing of average turnaround times for when the provider will respond to messages • Detailing of days, times, and circumstances when the provider will not respond to messages • Detailing of the best ways the patient can reach the provider in an emergency • Indication that asynchronous messages may be delayed or not received
Troubleshooting	• Description of the procedures for troubleshooting if the videoconferencing equipment is not working • Indication that a copy of the informed consent will be provided to the patient and include a list of alternatives and suggestions in case of equipment failure, accident, catastrophe, or natural disaster
Administrative	• Detailing of attendance expectations • Detailing of billing arrangements such as fees, when charged, and how charged • Detailing of billing practices for what is considered a late cancellation, no-show, or no-charge

involving medical care or law enforcement. Unfortunately, a lag in response time, or potentially no response if the provider is unable to establish pertinent information for the patient, has the potential to result in negative outcomes. To ensure safety throughout the use of the videoconferencing, it is suggested that the provider preventatively plan for crises at the onset of services. As adapted from work by Luxton and colleagues (2016, chap. 3) and Shore and Lu (2015), safety planning should occur in five broadly defined primary steps. First, a provider should determine the appropriateness of a patient for videoconferencing. Second, a provider should evaluate the appropriateness of the provider's and patient's available technology to meet the needs of the services. Third, the provider should critically evaluate the patient's location in which they will receive care, including any supports (e.g., family, friends, community organizations) they may have in the immediate area. Fourth, the provider should develop an emergency contact list and plan that is included in the patient's record. Fifth, and finally, the provider should create a step-by-step plan detailing expectations. When broken into more detail, as adapted by work by Luxton and colleagues (2016, chap. 3), the safety plan should have eight primary components: (a) the location address, phone number, and email address for the patient; (b) alternative emergency contacts of spouses, family members, friends, or local community members that may be able to assist during an emergency situation (i.e., names, addresses, phone numbers, emails); (c) the name, address, and phone number for the nearest medical center; (d) the name, address, and phone number for the nearest law enforcement office; (e) the criteria for what is considered an emergency situation versus a "write down and we'll talk about it at our next session" event; (f) the steps to make the environment safe if risk presents including the removal of alcohol, weapons, and other hazardous materials; (g) a step-by-step plan for what to do if the provider is available to speak to; and (h) a step-by-step plan for what to do if the provider is not available to speak to. While this information is suggested to be built into the informed consent forms (i.e., as part of the forms or added as a secondary emergency contact form that is a supplement to the primary informed consent forms), whether it is or is not, such information should be reviewed verbally and provided in writing. It is also suggested that regardless of whether a provider may be able to legally break continentality for an emergency situation, they secure release of information forms for the listed nonmedical and non-law enforcement contacts so that they may communicate with them as needed. Copies of the documents should be placed into the patient's medical record for easy access, with copies being provided to the patient. Finally, the provider should document that the plan was discussed, and the patient both understood and agreed. As sometimes patients may not provide the most complete information, it may also be wise to include a clause in the forms indicating that the provider or a representative of the organization may look up supplied information to verify correctness of the medical and law enforcement office (Lustgarten & Elhai, 2018). See Figure 4.3 for a sample template of an emergency contact information form.

While crises may be the most obvious reason to safety plan, the patient may also experience events during session that make them feel uncomfortable or unsafe, and desiring of an immediate stop to the videoconferencing. Unfortunately, some patients may be unable to vocalize this request in the moment. For instance, a patient may not have told a spouse or other family member that they are receiving psychological services due to a fear of stigma, legal challenges (e.g., custody battles), or a potentially abusive relationship. If during session, the patient directly says that they want to end the call, or if the provider continues talking while others can overhear the subject matter, such events can inadvertently disclose the therapeutic relationship. Regardless of the situation, it is important that the patient feels that they have a level of control to ensure a perception of safety and comfort. As such, it is suggested that the patient and provider collaboratively create a safety word or phrase. This word or phrase would be a cue for the provider to immediately end session without a required reason why. As an example, one could

Patient Telehealth Information Form

Prior to telehealth services being rendered, this form must be completed. A copy will be provided to the patient/family, as well as placed into the patient's medical record. Provided information must be accurate, may be verified by the provider or another appointed designee through the organization, and will be utilized to ensure the safety of all parties. If the treating provider determines there is a justifiable reason to break confidentiality to ensure the safety of the patient or another person due to the patient's behavior, the provider is authorized to do so. Conditions for breaking confidentiality may include, but are not limited to: if the patient is determined to be an active harm to themselves or to another, if abuse is recognized, or for a medical or behavioral emergency. If confidentiality must be broken, the treating provider will make reasonable efforts to inform the patient/parents prior to or following the disclosure, as allowed.

General Contact Information:

Patient name:	_____	Best email:	_____
Legal guardian name:	_____	Relationship to patient:	_____
Patient home address:	_____	Best phone number to reach patient or guardian:	_____

Emergency Contact Information:

Best alternative contact person 1:	_____	Relationship to patient	_____
		Best phone number to reach:	_____
Best alternative contact person 2:	_____	Relationship to patient	_____
		Best phone number to reach:	_____
Nearest medical center name:			_____
Nearest medical center address:	_____	Phone number:	_____
Nearest police department name:	_____		_____
Nearest police department address:	_____	Phone number:	_____

Figure 4.3 Sample emergency contact form*.

Note: *The sample information, especially the "Emergency Plan" section, will require additional tailored detail.

Please See Reverse for Additional Information

Emergency Plan:

- **If there is no fear of harm to patient or another person,** the patient/family is asked to write down information to be discussed at the next session. Should more immediate responses be required, the patient/family may call or email the provider. Depending on the nature of the information, the provider may require either a brief phone meeting, or an additional session to manage situations. If the provider deems email appropriate, an encrypted email client will be used.
- **If there appears to be a possibility of harm to the patient or to another person,** the patient/family is to immediately go to the local medical center/emergency room listed on this form. They are asked to contact the provider after safety has been ensured. If the patient/family is closer to another medical center than what is listed, they are to go to that location. Following stabilization and discharge, the patient/family is to provide the provider with an indication of what led to the need for a hospital visit, details of the hospital stay (e.g., medications, diagnoses, treatment summary), and both emotional and behavioral status post-discharge.
- **Note: At any time, the provider can decide that telehealth services are no longer appropriate and as such, may be terminated. If such an event occurs, the provider will provide alternative referral options should face-to-face treatment not be possible.**

Patient printed name:

Patient signature: _____

Parent/legal guardian printed name: _____

Parent/legal guardian signature: _____

Provider printed name: _____

Provider signature: _____

Figure 4.3 Cont.

use the word "banana" as their word in the context of individual therapy. Perhaps the patient had not disclosed that they were receiving therapy and did not want others to know. During session, the patient's significant other arrives home early and is already in distance to hear what is being discussed. The patient can then indicate, "I'm pretty hungry, I think I am going to go eat a banana" or "I really want a banana, gotta go," to immediately inform the provider that they should end the session. The provider can then immediately say "goodbye" and end the videoconferencing call. Alternatively, the provider and patient can agree that the provider would say a bit more, such as "I'm having some issues with the video/audio connection, I'll just talk to you later," to make it seem more friendly. Ultimately, having a code word or phrase can create an additional level of comfort for the patient without having to draw extra attention to the therapy itself.

Data Security: HIPAA

In efforts to protect the videoconferencing session, as well as any documentation arising from the clinical work, providers must be knowledgeable of data security protocols. Security regulations and laws vary by location. For example, the General Data Protection Regulation (GDPR) directs practice within the European Union (EU); and the Personal Information Protection and Electronic Document Act (PIPEDA), or a similar province/territory-specific legislation, guides private-sector providers within Canada. Specific to the United States, HIPAA guides professional work. As expanded and finalized in accordance with the HITECH Act through what was termed the Omnibus Rule, HIPAA has four primary rules applicable to videoconferencing: (a) Privacy Rule, (b) Security Rule, (c) Enforcement Rule, and (d) Breach Notification Rule. Combined rules are implemented to govern and ensure the privacy of a patient's PHI, whether physical or electronic (i.e., e-PHI). Related to the use of technology in clinical practice, protected information can include, but is not limited to, the patient's name, address, phone numbers, fax numbers, email addresses, social security numbers, medical record numbers, health plan beneficiary number, web addresses containing names or personal information, biometric identifiers such as fingerprints or vocal prints, full-face photos, or unique identifying numbers or codes (Sivilli, 2018b). HIPAA regulations apply to any covered entity. Per the US Health and Human Services (HHS, 2013g), covered entities include health plans, healthcare clearinghouses, and healthcare providers who conduct certain financial and administrative transactions electronically. Thus, under most circumstances, psychological providers can be considered a covered entity. The following is a summary of HIPAA rules and applications. Providers are encouraged to review the full guidelines presented on the HHS website (https://HHS.gov).

Privacy Rule

The Privacy Rule serves two primary functions. First, it allows patients access to their PHI. It also defines and limits the circumstances in which an individual's PHI may be used or disclosed by covered entities (HHS, 2013f). As such, the rule requires covered entities to enact privacy policies and procedures, to designate privacy officials responsible for developing and implementing the policies, to train any individual who comes into contact with the protected information, to mitigate any challenges, and to safeguard data. To fully comply with this rule for telepsychology, providers may have to redesign their policies and procedures, as well as update the training of any team members, to ensure understanding of how e-PHI may differ from traditional PHI.

Security Rule

The Security Rule protects a subset of information covered by the Privacy Rule, focusing on e-PHI (HHS, 2013g). Broadly defined by HHS (2013g), the rule ensures that covered entities must ensure the confidentiality, integrity, and availability of all e-PHI they create, receive, maintain, or transmit; identify and protect against reasonably anticipated threats to the security or integrity of the information; protect against reasonably anticipated, impermissible uses or disclosure; and ensure compliance by their workforce. To conform to the Security Rule, providers must enact standards for physical, administrative, and technical safeguards (HHS, 2013g).

Physical Safeguards

Physical safeguards involve the provider ensuring the security of the physical components of any PHI, physical or electronic. This includes having restricted access to not just the premises of the technology utilized for the videoconferencing and documentation, but also controlled access to the technology itself. This may include governing access to computers in a provider's office, or restricting access to a business laptop within their home (e.g., children cannot play games on it). Such protections can be as simple as basic locks on doors and placing laptops or other smaller technology in locked cabinets, or more complex means such as biometric devices (e.g., fingerprint scanners) for entering specific spaces or to use certain technology.

Administrative Safeguards

Administrative safeguards include ensuring the competence of all providers or staff members that will have access to the e-PHI. Competence can relate to both the use of, and proper storage of, any e-PHI, as well as legally acceptable reasons to disclose the information. Efforts to enforce this rule may include formal staff training, as well as ongoing monitoring and self-audits of efforts. Providers should also consider regular updates to ensure ongoing compliance. To monitor such activities, the provider can document the trainings in terms of when it was received, what topics it covered, and where it came from (e.g., specialized training from third-party organization, inter-company training as based on guiding organization literature).

Technical Safeguards

Technical safeguards include proper cybersecurity measures for the e-PHI. While there are no universal guidelines for cybersecurity, the National Institute of Standards and Technology (NIST) and the

National Cybersecurity Center of Excellence (NCCoE) created a US government-approved stance paper on privacy and security risks applicable to telepsychological practices, including videoconferencing (Arbelaez et al., 2018). The guidance suggests several specific security measures, including personal and network firewalls for systems, wireless access point routers that give the provider full network access control (i.e., the provider chooses who can gain access to the network), automated risk detection and prevention systems, and application security in the form of passwords and encryption. To more specifically guide practice, the stance paper detailed specifics for both the passwords and encryption. Passwords were suggested to be a minimum of eight characters and a combination of letters, numbers, and wild characters. It was suggested that providers avoid the use of password hints or writing the password down on paper, instead opting for a password locker program that can securely and digitally house all passwords for different applications. Encryption is a method of converting regular text and data into encoded information. This process essentially makes the information "unusable, unreadable, or indecipherable to unauthorized individuals" through "an algorithmic process to transform data into a form in which there is a low probability of assigning meaning without use of a confidential process or key" (HHS, 2013c). This means that once encrypted, the user requires a "key" to decrypt the information, recoding it back to an understandable format. As defined by the HHS, while the use of encryption is not specifically mandatory for the Security Rule if the rules can be met without use of encryption (HHS, 2013d), the use of advanced encryption standards (AES) is nonetheless highly recommended by both HHS and field experts to ensure that e-PHI practices adhere to the Security Rule (NIST, 2001; Yellowlees et al., 2010). More specifically, HHS suggests adhering to NIST and NCCoE standards of a minimum of 128-bit data encryption (NIST, 2001). As detailed by Arora (2012), when implemented properly and if the system is not already compromised due to a virus or another issue, AES of 128-bit or higher would take "at least 1 billion years for a supercomputer to breach." See Table 4.5 for a list of products indicating HIPAA-compliant encryption standards for data.

As providers utilizing videoconferencing often utilize third-party products (e.g., videoconferencing platforms, billing services) that will have access to e-PHI, the Security Rule also discusses the need for an executed business associate's agreement (BAA) with the utilized vendors (HHS, 2013g). A BAA is a contract between a covered entity (i.e., provider or provider organization) and the business associate (i.e., a person or organization other than a member of the covered entity who performs functions or activities on behalf of the covered entity and has access to e-PHI; HHS, 2013a). For example, a provider can have a BAA with a HIPAA-compliant videoconferencing platform company, email suites, or messaging programs. The BAA serves as an agreement that the business associate will follow HIPAA rules to protect the e-PHI. Further, it assists

Table 4.5 Products indicating HIPAA-compliant levels of encryption for data

Type	Options indicating HIPAA compliance
• Email	• Google Suites • Protonmail • Hush • Barracuda Email Security • Cryptshare
• Documents/drives	• Axcrypt • Veracrypt • Microsoft OneDrive • Symantec Endpoint Encryption
• Programs to share documents	• Dropbox • Box
• Phone messaging	• OhMD • TigerText • Zinc • QliqSoft • Notifyd • Spok Mobile

in protecting the provider and their practice from liability in the event of a data breach associated with or caused by the business associate vendor (HHS, 2013a).

Enforcement Rule

The Enforcement Rule has two primary purposes (HHS, 2017). First, it establishes procedures for investigations and hearings of those engaging in HIPAA violations. Second, it sets tiered civil penalties for the violations (HHS, 2013b). The first tier applies if the entity "did not know," resulting in a $100–$50,000 fine per violation. The second tier involves "reasonable cause," resulting in a $1,000–$50,000 fine per violation. The third tier involves "willful neglect" that was corrected, resulting in a $10,000–$50,000 fine per violation. Finally, the fourth tier involves "willful neglect" that was not corrected, resulting in a $50,000 fine per violation. Of note, while fines can vary as based upon several factors including if the covered entity exercised reasonable diligence to protect the information, fines are not to exceed $1,500,000 for identical violations during a calendar year (January 1 through the following December 31; Amount of a Civil Money Penalty, 2010).

Breach Notification Rule

The Breach Notification Rule sets standards for how and when breaches of unsecure PHI, physical or electronic, must be reported to the HHS (HHS, 2013e). This rule is especially pertinent to videoconferencing providers, as surveys in 2019 concluded that only approximately 72 percent of healthcare organizations conform to the HIPAA Security Rule, with only approximately 47 percent utilizing NIST-recommended security standards (CynergisTek, 2019). Common breaches have been indicated to include stolen or lost devices (e.g., laptop, smartphone), leaving technology accessible to unauthorized individuals, burglary at the office involving the hardware, unauthorized access to the technological systems, security threats (e.g., hacking), data breach caused by a third-party vendor, and incorrectly sending e-PHI to the wrong person (HIPAA Journal, 2019; Sivilli, 2018a). While the HHS provides guidance on informing them of breaches affecting either more than or less than 500 individuals on their website (www.hhs.gov/hipaa/for-professionals/breach-notification/breach-reporting/index.html), the American Psychological Association Practice Organization (2013) provided a detailed step-by-step plan that providers can follow, should a data breach occur. The three-step plan begins with a formal risk assessment. In this step, the provider should evaluate the nature and extent of the information involved in the breach, including to whom the information may have been disclosed to, whether it was actually acquired or viewed, and how the risk has been mitigated. Following this assessment, the provider should give notice to the patients affected. This notice should be provided in plain language, and include the provider's contact information, as well as a brief description of the breach including the following: dates; the types of protected information involved; steps the patient should take to protect against potential harm; and a brief description of steps the provider has taken to investigate the incident, mitigate harm, and protect against further breaches. Finally, as indicated by the HHS, a formal HHS report should be made.

Additional Considerations for Videoconferencing

In supplement of aforementioned ethical and legal considerations that should be considered prior to beginning the use of videoconferencing, once the provider begins services, they should enact several additional procedures to foster ongoing ethical and legal practice. More specifically, at the onset of each session, the provider should briefly verify the identity of the patient. This is especially important for those beginning videoconferencing services without having seen the patient in a F2F session. While identity verification may become less important as sessions progress (i.e., the provider recognizes the patient's appearance and voice), it is still a suggested strategy that can add an extra layer of security, especially in situations in which an individual may attempt to impersonate another (e.g., legal situations). One of the easiest means of identifying a patient's identity is to have them hold up a photo identification (e.g., license, passport) to the video camera.

In addition to verifying the patient's identity, in order to ensure that the provider remains informed, they should ask the patient if anyone else is in the videoconferencing room and will be participating in the session. As it is common for some patients to include family members, spouses, friends, community members, or children in sessions, it would be prudent for the provider to directly ask about this possibility before beginning and discussing anything confidential. This remains true even if the provider has no concerns with other members being present or participating.

Finally, the provider should ask about the patient's location, even if the location appears similar from session to session. This can help ensure that the provider does not practice in an unlicensed location. This is especially true if the patient often switches rooms in a home, is prone to having sessions in different locations due to a need to secure privacy or adapt to demands (e.g., work schedules not allowing the patient to return home), or travels for work (e.g., travels across states or countries, lives on a state line and goes short distances between two states for work).

Summary Points

- A provider's license and associated jurisdiction should be considered when offering videoconferencing, especially if one is to practice across state lines. Depending on jurisdiction, a provider may be liable in both locations should an issue or emergency arise.
- While varying by state, cross-state practice is often possible through temporary provisions (i.e., ≤ 30 days).
- Ongoing cross-state practice is possible through a provider becoming licensed in each state of practice, or enrolling in an interjurisdiction compact (e.g., PSYPACT) that makes them eligible to practice in any state entered into the compact without the need for additional licenses.
- Prior to the onset of videoconferencing, providers should critically evaluate patients for appropriateness. Particular consideration should be given to the patient's medical and mental health histories, diagnostic presentation, technical ability, technology availability, current levels of motivation, financial factors, and both location and transportation issues.
- Videoconferencing-specific informed consent should be secured both verbally and in writing above and beyond any standard informed consent process for F2F services. The process should detail aspects of practice, including standards of care, strengths and limitations, differences from F2F care, and administrative differences related to scheduling, communication, and billing.
- Prior to the onset of treatment, the provider should create a safety plan that includes a list of emergency contact information (e.g., names, addresses, emails, phone numbers) for both the patient and alternative individuals (e.g., spouse, family, friends, community members). Emergency contact information should also include the names, addresses, and phone numbers for the nearest medical center and law enforcement offices.

- Related to HIPAA, the provider should take care to ensure data security of any PHI, whether physical and electronic. For e-PHI, a provider should enact physical, technical, and administrative safeguards, including at least 128-bit encryption for data, training for anyone coming into contact with the information, appointment of a privacy official, and BAAs for any third-party vendors who will have access to the e-PHI.
- Should a data breach occur, the provider should critically evaluate the situation to determine the types and amounts of data breached, who the breach could affect, and how the breach was mitigated. The provider should then inform the patient(s) in plain language with detail of what occurred and what was done. Finally, the same information should be provided to HHS.
- At the onset of each session, the provider should verify the identity and location of the patient.

References

American Counseling Association (ACA). (n.d.). *Licensure requirements for professional counselors, a state by state report.* Retrieved from www.counseling.org/knowledge-center/licensure-requirements.

American Psychological Association (APA). (2020, March). *Informed consent checklist for telepsychological services.* Retrieved from www.apa.org/practice/programs/dmhi/research-information/informed-consent-checklist.

American Psychological Association Practice Organization. (2013). *The HIPAA final rule: What you need to know – guidance and privacy notice updates for psychologists.* Retrieved from www.apaservices.org/practice/update/2013/07-25/hipaa-final-rule.pdf.

American Telemedicine Association (ATA). (2003). *Home telehealth clinical guidelines.* Retrieved from www.americantelemed.org/resources/home-telehealth-clinical-guidelines/.

Amount of a Civil Money Penalty, 45 C.F.R. §160.404. (2010). Retrieved from www.govinfo.gov/app/details/CFR-2010-title45-vol1/CFR-2010-title45-vol1-sec160-404/summary.

Arbelaez, A., Daldos, R., Littlefield, K., Wang, S., & Weitzel, D. (2018). *Securing telehealth remote patient monitoring ecosystem: Cybersecurity for the telehealth sector (Draft).* Computer Security Resource Center. Retrieved from https://csrc.nist.gov/publications/detail/white-paper/2018/11/19/securing-telehealth-remote-patient-monitoring-ecosystem/draft.

Arora, M. (2012, May 7). How secure is AES against brute force attacks? *EE Times.* Retrieved from www.eetimes.com/how-secure-is-aes-against-brute-force-attacks/#.

Association of State and Provincial Psychology Boards (ASPPB). (2016). *PSYPACT legislative resource kit.* Retrieved from https://cdn.ymaws.com/asppb.site-ym.com/resource/resmgr/PSYPACT_Docs/PSYPACT_Resource_Kit_2.11.20.pdf.

Association of State and Provincial Psychology Boards (ASPPB). (2020). *Mobility program: Policies and procedures – v. 2.2020*. Retrieved from https://cdn.ymaws.com/www.asppb.net/resource/resmgr/asppb_mobility_program_polic.pdf.

Backhaus, A., Agha, Z., Maglione, M. L., Repp, A., Ross, B., Zuest, D., ... Thorp, S. R. (2012). Videoconferencing psychotherapy: A systematic review. *Psychological services, 9*(2), 111–131. https://doi.org/10.1037/a0027924.

Berryhill, M. B., Culmer, N., Williams, N., Halli-Tierney, A., Betancourt, A., Roberts, H., & King, M. (2019). Videoconferencing psychotherapy and depression: A systematic review. *Telemedicine and e-Health, 25*(6), 435–446. https://doi.org/10.1089/tmj.2018.0058.

Bischoff, R. J., Hollist, C. S., Smith, C. W., & Flack, P. (2004). Addressing the mental health needs of the rural underserved: Findings from a multiple case study of a behavioral telehealth project. *Contemporary Family Therapy, 26*(2), 179–198. https://doi.org/10.1023/B:COFT.0000031242.83259.fa.

Campbell, L. F., & Norcross, J. C. (2018). Do you see what we see? Psychology's response to technology in mental health. *Clinical Psychology: Science and Practice, 25*(2), e12237. https://doi.org/10.1111/cpsp.12237.

CynergisTek. (2019). *Measuring progress: Expanding the horizon*. Retrieved from https://insights.cynergistek.com/reports/2019-healthcare-cybersecurity-privacy-report.

Collie, K. R. (2004). Interpersonal communication in behavioral telehealth: What can we learn from other fields? In J. W. Bloom & G. R. Walz (Eds.), *Cybercounseling & cyberlearning: An encore* (pp. 345–365). Washington, DC: CAPS Press.

DeFife, J. A., & Hilsenroth, M. J. (2011). Starting off on the right foot: Common factor elements in early psychotherapy process. *Journal of Psychotherapy Integration, 21*(2), 172–191. https://doi.org/10.1037/a0023889.

Drum, K. B., & Littleton, H. L. (2014). Therapeutic boundaries in telepsychology: Unique issues and best practice recommendations. *Professional Psychology: Research and Practice, 45*(5), 309–315. https://doi.org/10.1037/a0036127.

Duncan, A. B., Velasquez, S. E., & Nelson, E-L. (2014). Using videoconferencing to provide psychological services to rural children and adolescents: A review and case example. *Journal of Clinical Child & Adolescent Psychology, 43*(1), 115–127. https://doi.org/10.1080/15374416.2013.836452.

Feijt, M. A., de Kort, Y. A., Bongers, I. M., & IJsselsteijn, W. A. (2018). Perceived drivers and barriers to the adoption of eMental health by psychologists: The construction of the levels of adoption of eMental health model. *Journal of Medical Internet Research, 20*(4), e153. https://doi.org/10.2196/jmir.9485.

Gupta, A., & Sao, D. (2011). The constitutionality of current legal barriers to telemedicine in the United States: Analysis and future directions of its relationship to national and international health care reform. *Health Matrix, 21*, 385–442.

Henry, B. W., Block, D. E., Ciesla, J. R., McGowan, B. A., & Vozenilek, J. A. (2017). Clinician behaviors in telehealth care delivery: A systematic review. *Advances in Health Sciences Education, 22*(4), 869–888. https://doi.org/10.1007/s10459-016-9717-2.

Hidy, B., Porch, E., Reed, S., Parish, M. B., & Yellowlees, P. (2013). Social networking and mental health. In K. Myers & C. L. Turvey (Eds.), *Telemental health: Clinical, technical, and administrative foundations for evidence-based practice* (pp. 367–395). London: Elsevier.

HIPAA Journal. (2019, April 26). The most common HIPAA violations you should be aware of. Retrieved from www.hipaajournal.com/common-hipaa-violations/.

Hochhauser, M. (2007). Consent forms: No easy read. *Applied Clinical Trials*, *16*(5), 74.

Huggins, R. (2016). Using mobile phone communication for therapeutic intervention. In S. Goss, K. Anthony, L. S. Stretch, & D. M. Nagel (Eds.), *Technology in mental health: Applications in practice, supervision, and training* (2nd ed., pp. 28–42). Springfield, IL: Charles C. Thomas.

Jacobs, J. A. (n.d.). Informed consent for telepsychology. Trust Parma. Retrieved from https://parma.trustinsurance.com/Portals/0/documents/Sample%20 Informed%20Consent%20for%20Telepsychology.docx.

Johns Hopkins Medicine. (2016). *Informed consent guidance: How to prepare a readable consent form.* Retrieved from www.hopkinsmedicine.org/institutional_ review_board/guidelines_policies/guidelines/informed_consent_ii.html.

Koocher, G. P., & Morray, E. (2000). Regulation of telepsychology: A survey of state attorneys general. *Professional Psychology: Research and Practice*, *31*(5), 503–508. https://doi.org/10.1037//0735-7028.31.5.503.

Kramer, G. M., Mishkind, M. C., Luxton, D. D., & Shore, J. H. (2013). Managing risk and protecting privacy in telemental health: An overview of legal, regulatory and risk management issues. In K. Myers & C. L. Turvey (Eds.), *Telemental health: Clinical, technical, and administrative foundations for evidence-based practice* (pp. 83–108). London: Elsevier.

Lehman, J., & Phelps. S. (Eds.). (2005). *West's encyclopedia of American law* (2nd ed.). Detroit, MI: Thomson Gale.

Lustgarten, S. D., & Elhai, J. D. (2018). Technology use in mental health practice and research: Legal and ethical risks. *Clinical Psychology: Science and Practice*, *25*(2), e12234. https://doi.org/10.1111/cpsp.12234.

Luxton, D. D., Nelson, E. -L., & Maheu, M. M. (2016). *A practitioner's guide to telemental health: How to conduct legal, ethical and evidence-based telepractice.* Washington, DC: American Psychological Association.

Martin, E. A. (Ed.). (2003). *Oxford dictionary of law.* Oxford: Oxford University Press.

Meyers, L. (2020, April 8). Interstate compact plan provides hope for licensure portability. *Counseling Today*. Retrieved from https://ct.counseling.org/2020/04/ interstate-compact-plan-provides-hope-for-licensure-portability/.

Muoio, D. (2017, October 18). Nearly every state has updated its telehealth legislation since last year. *Mobi Health News*. Retrieved from www.mobihealthnews.com/content/report-nearly-every-state-has-updated-its-telehealth-legislation-last-year.

Murphy, J. M., & Pomerantz, A. M. (2016). Informed consent: An adaptable question format for telepsychology. *Professional Psychology: Research and Practice*, *47*(5), 330–339. https://doi.org/10.1037/pro0000098.

National Institute of Standards and Technology (NIST). (2001). *Federal Information Processing Standards Publication 197: Announcing the advanced encryption standard (AES)*. Retrieved from https://nvlpubs.nist.gov/nistpubs/ FIPS/NIST.FIPS.197.pdf.

Oldham, M., Kellett, S., Miles, E., & Sheeran, P. (2012). Interventions to increase attendance at psychotherapy: A meta-analysis of randomized controlled trials. *Journal of Consulting and Clinical Psychology*, *80*(5), 928–939. https://doi. org/10.1037/a0029630.

Perle, J. G., Langsam, L. C., & Nierenberg, B. (2011). Controversy clarified: An updated review of clinical psychology and tele-health. *Clinical Psychology Review*, *31*(8), 1247–1258. https://doi.org/10.1016/j.cpr.2011.08.003.

Perle, J. G., & Nierenberg, B. (2013). How psychological telehealth can alleviate society's mental health burden: A literature review. *Journal of Technology in Human Services*, *31*(1), 22–41. https://doi.org/10.1080/15228835.2012.760332.

Reardon, M. L., Cukrowicz, K. C., Reeves, M. D., & Joiner, T. E. (2002). Duration and regularity of therapy attendance as predictors of treatment outcome in an adult outpatient population. *Psychotherapy Research*, *12*(3), 273–285. https://doi.org/10.1080/713664390.

Shore, P., & Lu, M. (2015). Patient safety planning and emergency management. In P. W. Tuerk & P. Shore (Eds.), *Clinical videoconferencing in telehealth: Program development and practice* (pp. 167–201). Cham: Springer International.

Sivilli, F. (2018a, July 6). Common HIPAA violations to avoid. Telebehavioral Health Institute. Retrieved from https://telehealth.org/blog/common-hipaa-violation/.

Sivilli, F. (2018b, May 19). Developing your basic HIPAA checklist. Telebehavioral Health Institute. Retrieved from https://telehealth.org/blog/basic-hipaa-checklist/.

Suler, J. (2004). The online disinhibition effect. *Cyberpsychology & Behavior*, *7*(3), 321–326. https://doi.org/10.1089/1094931041291295.

Tamariz, L., Palacio, A., Robert, M., & Marcus, E. N. (2013). Improving the informed consent process for research subjects with low literacy: A systematic review. *Journal of General Internal Medicine*, *28*(1), 121–126. https://doi.org/10.1007/s11606-012-2133-2.

Tryon, G. S., & Winograd, G. (2011). Goal consensus and collaboration. *Psychotherapy*, *38*(4), 385–289. https://doi.org/10.1037/a0022061.

Turvey, C. L. (2018). Telemental health care delivery: Evidence base and practical considerations. In J. J. Magnavita (Ed.), *Using technology in mental health practice* (pp. 25–42). Washington, DC: American Psychological Association.

US Food & Drug Administration (FDA). (2014). *Informed consent: Draft guidance for IRBs, clinical investigators, and sponsors.* Retrieved from www.fda.gov/regulatory-information/search-fda-guidance-documents/informed-consent.

US Health and Human Services (HHS). (2013a). *Business associate contracts.* Retrieved from www.hhs.gov/hipaa/for-professionals/covered-entities/sample-business-associate-agreement-provisions/index.html.

US Health and Human Services (HHS). (2013b). *Federal register: Part II.* Retrieved from www.govinfo.gov/content/pkg/FR-2013-01-25/pdf/2013-01073.pdf.

US Health and Human Services (HHS). (2013c). *Guidance to render unsecure protected health information unusable, unreadable, or indecipherable to unauthorized individuals.* Retrieved from www.hhs.gov/hipaa/for-professionals/breach-notification/guidance/index.html.

US Health and Human Services (HHS). (2013d). *Is the use of encryption mandatory in the Security Rule?* Retrieved from www.hhs.gov/hipaa/for-professionals/faq/2001/is-the-use-of-encryption-mandatory-in-the-security-rule/index.html.

US Health and Human Services (HHS). (2013e). *Submitting notice of a breach to the secretary.* Retrieved from www.hhs.gov/hipaa/for-professionals/breach-notification/breach-reporting/index.html.

US Health and Human Services (HHS). (2013f). *Summary of the HIPAA Privacy Rule.* Retrieved from www.hhs.gov/hipaa/for-professionals/privacy/laws-regulations/index.html.

US Health and Human Services (HHS). (2013g). *Summary of the HIPAA Security Rule.* Retrieved from www.hhs.gov/hipaa/for-professionals/security/laws-regulations/index.html.

US Health and Human Services (HHS). (2017). *The HIPAA Enforcement Rule.* Retrieved from www.hhs.gov/hipaa/for-professionals/special-topics/enforcement-rule/index.html.

Yellowlees, P., Shore, J., & Roberts, L. (2010). Practice guidelines for videoconferencing telemental health, October 2009. *Telemedicine and e-Health, 16*(10), 1074–1089. https://doi.org/10.1089/tmj.2010.0148.

5 Videoconferencing Logistics
Overview

While videoconferencing services have garnered significant interest among both providers and patients, research and guiding organizations have suggested that positive outcomes are predominantly achieved when providers account for specific factors unique to the technology. Such factors can be grouped into two broad categories of practice: setting up the logistics of the videoconferencing and conducting the actual sessions.

Initial steps involve the providers reviewing logistical factors of the videoconferencing experience. Broadly categorized, primary logistical considerations include: (a) computer system, (b) video camera, (c) display screen, (d) microphone, (e) videoconferencing platform, (f) bandwidth and latency, and (g) room setup. Each factor both uniquely and collaboratively contributes to successful videoconferencing between a provider and a patient. While many providers may be familiar with the general notions of each consideration, proper utilization of videoconferencing requires them to consider the more minute details of the practices, as these particulars are what can foster success and prevent issues. Such details apply to the provider's location and technology, as well as those of the patient. Of note, while some patients may be able to set up all necessary components with little guidance, others may require more "hands-on" coaching and assistance in which the provider talks them through each step, with active testing at each stage. For example, the provider may have to coach the patient on how to set up a videoconferencing camera via telephone before testing the camera through the desired videoconferencing platform. While testing, the provider can educate the patient on what to click and what to avoid clicking to maximize the session.

Once the logistical factors have been fully detailed, set up, and problem-solved, at the onset of the care, the provider must review and implement structured plans for the actual conducting of the videoconferencing sessions. This plan should include a stepwise procedure beginning with the evaluation of the environment for appropriateness, testing of equipment, and the verification of locations and identities. Such plans should also account for difficulties, as well as means of fostering success during the actual sessions, including possible modifications for how a provider speaks or physically moves in order to emphasize key points and demonstrate empathetic responding.

The following chapters provide relatively brief, but detailed discussions for both procedural phases, beginning with an outline of the seven logistical considerations. This is followed by tips for video and audio to maximize the sessions. Next is a stepwise overview of setting up the videoconferencing and conducting the actual sessions. Finally, means of documenting the session content and processes are reviewed.

6 Videoconferencing Logistics
System Considerations

In order to ensure a successful videoconferencing process, before a provider even considers video or audio components, they must critically evaluate the systems. On a basic level, this evaluation is needed to ensure that both the provider and the patient's systems can manage the equipment and components needed. Fortunately, the proliferation of technology has created smaller, cheaper, more readily available, more powerful, and increasingly user-friendly systems that can be used for videoconferencing, whether it be completed through a computer, laptop, tablet, or smartphone system (to collectively be referred to as "computer"). In evaluating such components, the provider should consider both the hardware and software. The following is a simplified summary of key components that providers should consider for the systems used in videoconferencing.

Hardware Considerations

From a technical standpoint, to evaluate whether one's system can handle videoconferencing, they must ensure appropriate hardware. Hardware refers to the physical parts of a computer system, including the central processing unit (CPU), random access memory (RAM), graphics cards, sound card, mouse, and keyboard. While many components ensure a successful system, two worthy of highlighting as related to videoconferencing are the CPU and RAM.

CPU

The CPU, sometimes referred to as the processor, is one of the main components in making a system run and is essentially part of the brain of a computer (Encyclopaedia Britannica, 2018; Martindale, 2020a). More specifically, the CPU is a piece of hardware that allows a computer to interact with programs (i.e., software) to translate the data and create output that is presented on the user's display screen. The CPU manages everything from the computer's startup to the videoconferencing session itself. Ultimately, better CPUs allow for faster processing of information and thus faster computer functioning, while slower CPUs create slower processes and a worse user experience. Related to desktop and laptop computers, some of the most common CPUs include the Intel Core line of i3, i5, i7, or i9 processors. While each has differences in terms of specifications and features, for the purpose of the videoconferencing discussion, the larger the number of the processor, generally speaking, the more powerful and faster it will be. Nevertheless, providers do not necessarily need the "top-of-the-line" CPUs for videoconferencing. For example, while not all videoconferencing platforms indicate CPU specifications, Zoom, one of the more common videoconferencing platforms, details suggested specifications of an Intel Core i5 or higher CPU for a single-screen computer (Zoom, n.d.b).

RAM

Supplementing the CPU, RAM is hardware that allows a computer system to temporarily store short-term or working data (Encyclopaedia Britannica, 2009; Martindale, 2020b). While some videoconferencing platforms require a lot of memory, others do not. Regardless of how much data is used by the videoconferencing platform itself, systems constantly run other programs in the "background" (e.g., email, reminder programs, system updates, system security), potentially using RAM that is not known to the provider or patient. As such, evaluating the size of both the provider and patient's computer system's RAM becomes increasingly important. In combination with other hardware components, such as a CPU, the higher the amount of RAM, the faster computers generally run, and the more programs that can be simultaneously opened without slowing down the system. More specifically, limited RAM can cause a computer to move very slowly or lag. Related to videoconferencing, this can cause issues with seeing or hearing each other in real time (e.g., the patient freezing on video, gaps in audio). Unfortunately, there is no specific amount of RAM that is required to effectively run videoconferencing, as it varies by several factors beyond just the videoconferencing platform. For example, WebEx suggests at least two gigabytes of RAM along with an appropriate CPU to send or receive high-definition video (WebEx, n.d.). Alternatively, Zoom suggests at least four gigabytes of RAM along with an appropriate CPU (Zoom, n.d.a). Regardless of amount, providers should be aware of RAM as a potential influencing factor, should the videoconferencing program not be working properly (e.g., very slow performance).

Selecting Hardware

While no universal standards exist for videoconferencing, if one has computer hardware from the last several years (e.g., Intel i5 was introduced in 2009; Intel, n.d.), it is likely powerful enough to facilitate a high-definition videoconferencing call. Nevertheless, as there are numerous factors that go into whether the videoconferencing platforms will work on one's hardware, the simplest and most time-effective technique is to merely attempt to install and run the components on the computer system and see how it works. If unsuccessful, the provider can evaluate the CPU and RAM before potentially gaining consultation from more tech-savvy individuals in efforts to more clearly establish reasons for issues. Should a system merely be insufficient (i.e., older CPU, too little RAM), the user may need to gain access to one that is more suitable.

Software Considerations

Complementing the hardware is the computer software, or the programs that are put on and used by the computer systems. Many aspects of software should be considered. First and foremost is the computer's operating system (OS), which can include Microsoft Windows, iOS, and Linux, among others. Further, each OS has different versions (e.g., Microsoft Windows Vista, Windows 7, Windows 10), with each coming with new updates. The OS is not only important due to some videoconferencing platforms requiring specific versions to run at all, but also to ensure the compatibility with certain internet browsers, such as the popular Chrome, Safari, and Internet Explorer, which are often required to run browser-based videoconferencing platforms (i.e., running the videoconferencing from the internet browser without having to download additional programs to the computer). While many platforms have both downloadable and browser-based versions, some patients may not want to download additional software to their computer if not needed. This is especially true if their computer is already running slower than desired. As such, evaluating both the provider's and patient's OS and browsers can help prevent later issues with the software of choice, or if the videoconferencing platform must be unexpectedly changed due to technical issues with the primary selected program.

While a computer's OS is important for running software, it is also important for security reasons. Updated versions of the OS often improve the computer system's firewall. This firewall is a form of network security controlling data coming in and out of one's computer system, as based upon set rules. Essentially, it is governing the communication between the user's trusted system and the outside untrusted networks in efforts to protect against attacks to the user's computer network (Cisco, n.d.; Encyclopaedia Britannica, 2020). Although firewalls help improve security, they are only one part of needed protection for a videoconferencing provider. The provider should also evaluate their security software, and that of the patient. Not having adequate security places a computer system at risk of threats caused by malicious software, commonly referred to simply as malware. Malware is broadly defined as computer software designed to damage a computer system, or make it susceptible to others, thus placing the patient's e-PHI or other information on the infected computer at risk (ESET, n.d.; Norton, n.d.). Examples of malware can include computer viruses, adware, spyware, rootkits, or ransomware. To protect against malware, specialized security software should be installed on all computers used for the videoconferencing processes. While a provider cannot always control the patient's system, they can provide guidance on what types of antimalware software should be installed, as well as suggestions for what features a patient should look for. For example, one would desire real-time screening of data to protect from attacks that could come from visiting the wrong website, or clicking on an email link that the provider or patient thought was from a respectable source, but really attempted to install a malware program on the computer. In addition to real-time monitoring, the ability to schedule deep scans of the full computer system can be helpful. These scans can review the entire system, including both common and less accessed files, to ensure that the system is free from malware that could create problems or security threats. Further, they can be scheduled at times when they would not significantly interfere with one's work (i.e., some scans utilize significant RAM, thus increasing the potential for the computer to slow). While important features, none would be very useful if they did not have the most up-to-date malware definitions allowing for detection of the ever-increasing number of malicious programs. As such, having an antimalware program that has ongoing and frequent database updates is essential. Unfortunately, more features and better databases often require antimalware programs that are subscription-based, potentially precluding use for some patients who have financial restrictions. Nevertheless, if one is unable to purchase a higher-level package, there are many antimalware programs that are free, have tiers of subscription costs, and/or have frequent sales, making them more affordable options. While providers are encouraged to review the benefits and limitations of each possibility, common options include McAfee, Kaspersky, Bitdefender, Norton, Webroot SecureAnywhere, Avast, Malwarebytes, ESET, Microsoft Defender, and ZoneAlarm,

Restricting Access

While having appropriate security software is important, computers may still be susceptible to unauthorized access. As such, a provider should consider if the computers are private or accessible to others. This consideration is important for those who share the technology with colleagues, or allow their children or other family members to utilize them for entertainment purposes. Even if the computer system has powerful hardware, others can impair it by downloading unnecessary programs, or place it at risk by inadvertently downloading malware. As such, it is suggested that the computers used for videoconferencing be restricted as best as possible, and not used for general internet "surfing," to play games, or for other activities that are not professional in nature. It is also suggested that the computers are placed in locked areas to ensure physical safeguards.

For providers or patients who cannot physically restrict the computers, but still want to ensure the highest level of security and conformity with HIPAA, they can implement system-based features that limit access of the computer system to only authorized users. First, passwords can be required to log into the computer system itself (e.g., general password login to gain access to the desktop screen), and potentially implemented for individual programs. Password protection can be activated from most OS systems settings, including general password settings, in addition to the increasingly available parental lock programs. While predominantly intended to restrict child access, the parental locks can serve the same functions regardless of age, including restricting access without the primary user's password to unlock the features. Further, such programs can inform the primary user of others' activity and attempts to access aspects of the system that they have been restricted from. Should a provider or patient desire more specific, adaptable, or secure settings to suit their needs, third-party accessibility programs can be utilized.

To supplement passwords, the provider should consider the use of encryption programs of at least 128-bit or higher. Encryption programs can be used to encrypt specific files or folders, or entire disks (e.g., hard drives), meaning that one would need the "key" to decrypt the information (see Chapter 4 for more information on encryption). In doing so, even if a user gains access to the physical system, and can log in to the computer, they would still need to decrypt the system or file information with (ideally) a different password than what was used to log in before they are able to reasonable view or access the encrypted information. For a list of encryption programs for different types of data, please see Table 4.5.

Evaluating the CPU, RAM, and OS

Provided that not all providers may be aware of their computer specifications, there are easy ways to check the type of CPU, RAM, and OS version. Of note, there are multiple ways to find the same information, with only a few being described here. For Windows computers, a provider can left click the Windows icon on the bottom left of their display screen and either manually search for or type in "Control Panel." Once open, they should navigate to "System." Within this view, the "Windows edition" OS will be listed (e.g., Windows 10 Home), as well as the details of the CPU and RAM. Alternatively, a provider can right click on their bottom-left Windows icon and select "Task Manager." Once opened, they should navigate to the "Performance" tab, which will allow the provider to click on different options to see the specifications, including those related to the CPU and RAM. For Mac computers, a provider can go to the Apple menu on the top left of their display screen and select "About This Mac," which will show the OS, CPU, and RAM information. Alternatively, the provider can click the "Launchpad icon" in the dock area, then "Other," and finally "System Information."

Summary Points

- Evaluation of the computer systems that both the provider and patient will be using is essential to ensure smooth, appropriate, and secure videoconferencing processes.
- Computer hardware components to evaluate include the CPU and RAM. Assuming all other components are functioning properly (e.g., internet connection), a better processor and higher amount of RAM can facilitate a smoother videoconferencing session.
- Computer software components to evaluate include the OS and antimalware programs.
- Users should restrict access of the computer systems to unauthorized users through the use of physical safeguards (e.g., locking computers in safe locations), passwords, and encryption programs.

References

Cisco. (n.d.). What is a firewall? Retrieved from www.cisco.com/c/en/us/products/security/firewalls/what-is-a-firewall.html.

Encyclopaedia Britannica. (2009, March 13). RAM. Retrieved from www.britannica.com/technology/RAM-computing.

Encyclopaedia Britannica. (2018, March 14). Central processing unit. Retrieved from www.britannica.com/technology/central-processing-unit.

Encyclopaedia Britannica. (2020, May 7). Firewall. Retrieved from www.britannica.com/technology/firewall.

ESET. (n.d.). What is malware? www.eset.com/us/antimalware/.

Intel. (n.d.). Product specifications: advanced search. Retrieved from https://ark.intel.com/content/www/us/en/ark/search/featurefilter.html?productType=873&1_Filter-Family=122139.

Martindale, J. (2020a, April 14). What is a CPU? *Digital Trends*. Retrieved from www.digitaltrends.com/computing/what-is-a-cpu/.

Martindale, J. (2020b, March 15). What is RAM? *Digital Trends*. Retrieved from www.digitaltrends.com/computing/what-is-ram/.

Norton. (n.d.). What is malware and how can we prevent it? Retrieved from https://us.norton.com/internetsecurity-malware.html.

WebEx. (n.d.). Minimum system requirements for video conferencing. Retrieved from https://support.webex.com/webex/v1.3/mc/en_US/in_meeting/r_Minimum_system_requirements_for_video_conferencing.html.

Zoom. (n.d.a). System requirements for Windows, macOS, and Linux. Retrieved from https://support.zoom.us/hc/en-us/articles/201362023-System-requirements-for-Windows-macOS-and-Linux.

Zoom. (n.d.b). System requirements for Zoom rooms. Retrieved from https://support.zoom.us/hc/en-us/articles/204003179-System-Requirements-for-Zoom-Rooms#h_1a06a99f-46ff-4736-92ee-507ff12a4d4b.

7 Videoconferencing Logistics
Video Camera Considerations

One of the defining aspects of videoconferencing compared to other telepsychology modalities (e.g., telephone, email, texting, messaging programs) is the ability to see the patient in real time. To facilitate this, it is important that the provider and patient have adequate video cameras, sometimes referred to as web cameras. For the provider, this will allow for a clear view of both the patient's overt and more nuanced nonverbal behaviors that may be relevant to an assessment or treatment (e.g., tears in eyes, minor facial grimaces). Although financial considerations may prevent some patients from securing an optimal camera, the provider can still supply recommendations for what criteria is best in order to maximize the quality. Ultimately, whether set up as part of a larger institutional telepsychology system (e.g., a third-party company installs all technology), built into a preexisting computer system, or a plug-and-play USB camera, several specific features can be viewed as desirable for the videoconferencing cameras.

Desired Features

Easy to Install and Problem-Solve

On the simplest level, providers should seek and recommend cameras that are relatively easy to install and problem-solve (Spargo et al., 2013). This consideration is especially relevant to those who may be creating their own videoconferencing system without the help of a third-party organization who would install or provide technical support. Two of the simplest options for video cameras involve the provider or patient using either built-in cameras or seeking plug-and-play USB cameras. Built-in cameras may be available as part of a computer monitor, laptop, tablet, or smartphone. One of the perks of this method is that drivers and software are generally already installed onto the computer, making the use of the camera with the videoconferencing platform relatively seamless. Alternatively, as suggested in the name, plug-and-play USB cameras involve the provider or patient plugging the camera into an acceptable USB port, at which point the camera communicates with the computer system to automatically install any needed drivers or software, resulting in simple installation and immediate usage with videoconferencing platforms. Both methods can be viewed as relatively simple and cost-effective.

Camera Software

Many newer video cameras either come with specialized camera-specific software that is installed when the camera is plugged in (e.g., if plug-and-play USB), or can be downloaded from the camera company's website. While different cameras allow for different features and options, such software may allow the ability for a provider to customize the videoconferencing experience related to image quality, resolution, compression, and pan-tilt-zoom features.

Image Quality Settings

Some software packages allow for the provider to modify the image quality of the video cameras through specific settings. For example, assuming the camera has such functionality, software can allow the user to change the field of view of the camera itself, including between 65 and 90 degrees (Figure 7.1). On the lower end, 65 degrees would allow for a more limited view of the user and their environment unless they physically move the camera farther back. Contrastingly, a larger field of view, such as 90 degrees, would allow for the provider or patient to see a larger view of the other user and their environment, essentially lengthening the left and right sides of the visible area. A larger view may be especially helpful for multiple people participating in the videoconferencing session. The software may also allow for a user to toggle between either a manual or auto-focus feature. For providers who want the easiest possible solution for themselves and their patients, turning on the auto-focus option will allow the camera to focus on whatever is placed in front of it, whether the object moves forward or back. This can be especially helpful if the provider or patient holds objects (e.g., paperwork, videos on their phone) to the camera, requiring the camera to adjust from the larger view of the person to the object, and then back to the larger view without creating a blurred or disrupted image clarity. Also related to image quality, the camera software may have settings that allow for adjustment of brightness and contrast. Such features are important for providers or patients who may be in a setting where light changes due to windows, or if they are constantly changing locations for the videoconferencing sessions. If the image quality appears too bright, the user can manually lower the settings to make their image appear more visually appropriate for the other user. Similarly, contrast can be adjusted to more clearly differentiate the light and dark aspects of the image. Finally, some software packages include an anti-flicker setting, reducing the flickering that the user's camera detects from artificial lighting of a room (e.g., overhead lights), or from a background LCD screen (e.g., TV, computer display).

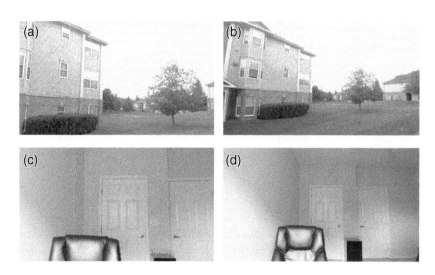

Figure 7.1 Examples of camera field of view: (a) 65-degree field of view; (b) 90-degree field of view; (c) 65-degree field of view; (d) 90-degree field of view.

Resolution Options

The resolution of the video will determine how clear the picture is for the other user. The level determines how many pixels the image contains, with pixels being the tiny squares that make up a digital image (Morris, 2019). As demonstrated in Figure 7.2, the higher the resolution, the larger the number of pixels, and the clearer the image becomes. Resolution can be presented in numerous ways, including lower to standard resolutions of 240p, 360p, and 480p, and higher resolutions, such as 720p, 1080p, 1440p, and 2160p (i.e., 4K; Google, n.d.). Although higher resolution means greater clarity, some systems and internet connections may not be able to smoothly run higher-resolution video quality without issues. For example, while a provider may have a 1080p camera and is transmitting the high-definition video image, the patient's system may be unable to smoothly run the high resolution, creating lag for them. To account for such issues, some cameras and associated software have settings to lower the resolution of the camera if needed. As such, higher-resolution cameras may have a maximum of 4K, but can be scaled down to 1440p, 1080, 720p, or 480p. For videoconferencing, while no universal standards exist, many have indicated that the services should be delivered at a resolution high enough to ensure the quality of the image for the care, similar to what would be observed in a F2F interaction (e.g., Shore et al., 2018). When one considers that high-definition video quality allows the provider and patient to see each other more clearly, and can facilitate easier identification of nonverbal behaviors, it is reasonable to suggest the use of 720p video quality or higher, as lower quality may not clearly demonstrate more subtle behaviors.

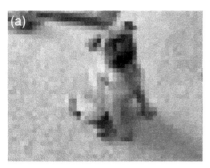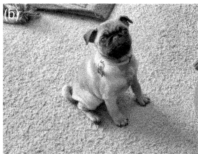

Figure 7.2 Example of the effects of resolution: (a) low resolution; (b) high resolution.

Compression Options

Complementing video resolution is video compression (Figure 7.3). Compression allows for images and video to consume less space. The higher the amount of compression, the more data is removed, and the worse the images or video appears compared to the original (Romero, 2018). In videoconferencing, higher compression can result in less detail in the images of both the provider and patient, thus reducing the ability to see more subtle changes (e.g., tears in eyes). As such, if available for the specific camera and software, the provider should consider the compression options, with the least amount of compression being applied as possible.

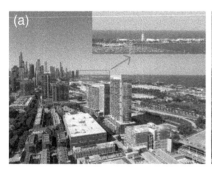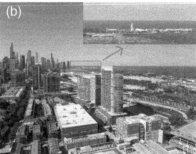

Figure 7.3 Example of the effects of compression with zoomed-in image: (a) original; (b) high compression.

Pan–Tilt–Zoom (PTZ)

While not a feature of all commercial video cameras, some higher-end cameras allow a provider to control a patient's camera's panning, tilting, and zooming features from a distance. As many videoconferencing sessions are structured in a way that shows the patient from the mid-waist and above, considerable nonverbal information may be lost. Alternatively, if the patient is instructed to sit farther back so that the provider can see a larger view of them, more discrete behaviors may be missed. The ability to pan, tilt, and zoom in real time can allow the provider to track a patient's movement (e.g., a patient is pacing, a child moves to a different location in the room), tilt the camera up or down to see different body parts (e.g., tilting lower to see if the patient is bouncing their legs or wringing their hands from anxiety), and zoom in on specific locations of the patient to view their response to presented information (e.g., zooming in on eyes to see if they are tearing). While not all have such functionality, some videoconferencing platforms have built-in controls for such cameras. For example, with appropriate cameras as determined by the specified videoconferencing platform, Zoom and VSee advertise far-end PTZ camera control which can give the provider access to a patient's PTZ camera (VSee, 2015; Zoom, n.d.). While some patients may be willing to purchase PTZ cameras for their sessions at the recommendation of their provider, providers may also consider purchasing a few of the desired cameras (e.g., can pan, tilt, or zoom silently) and loaning them to patients for the duration of their sessions. In this regard, the provider can mail the camera after the patient signs documentation agreeing to take care of the equipment and to send it back when the sessions are completed.

Summary Points

- Regardless of whether using a third-party company that installs an entire video camera system, adapting a preinstalled camera (e.g., laptop camera), or utilizing a plug-and-play USB camera, the provider should consider several aspects of the camera to ensure it is functional for their therapeutic needs.
- The cameras should be easy to install and problem-solve.
- Providers should seek cameras that have associated software to customize the video image quality. While varying by camera and software, such settings may include the field of view, focus, brightness, and contrast.
- The cameras should allow high-definition video resolution, ideally 720p or above.
- The camera software should allow for lower compression in order to ensure that significant image detail is not lost.

- If possible, a silent PTZ feature of the patient's camera can be helpful to track a patient and see behaviors that may not be readily available if the camera is in a fixed position.

References

Google. (n.d.). Video resolution and aspect ratios. YouTube Help. Retrieved from https://support.google.com/youtube/answer/6375112?co=GENIE. Platform%3DDesktop&hl=en.

Morris, K. O. (2019, December 20). The basics of image resolution. Vimeo Blog. Retrieved from https://vimeo.com/blog/post/the-basics-of-image-resolution/.

Romero, A. (2018, March 27). What is video encoding? Codecs and compression techniques. IBM. Retrieved from https://blog.video.ibm.com/streaming-video-tips/what-is-video-encoding-codecs-compression-techniques/.

Shore, J. H., Yellowlees, P., Caudill, R., Johnston, B., Turvey, C., Mishkind, M., … Hilty, D. (2018). Best practices in videoconferencing telemental health April 2018. *Telemedicine and e-Health*, *24*(11), 827–832. https://doi.org/10.1089/tmj.2018.0237.

Spargo, G., Karr, A., & Turvey, C. L. (2013). Technology options for the provision of mental health care through videoteleconferencing. In K. Myers & C. L. Turvey (Eds.), *Telemental health: Clinical, technical, and administrative foundations for evidence-based practice* (pp. 135–151). London: Elsevier.

VSee. (2015, October 5). VSee + PTZOptics remote PTZ camera control for telemedicine. Retrieved from https://vsee.com/blog/vsee-ptzoptics-remote-control-ptz-cameras-telemedicine/.

Zoom. (n.d.). Far-end camera control. Retrieved from https://support.zoom.us/hc/en-us/articles/203028599-Far-end-camera-control.

8 Videoconferencing Logistics
Display Screen Considerations

Even if users have a high-definition video camera for the videoconferencing sessions, consideration must also be given to the display screens that the images are displayed on. While some may think that having a larger screen, such as a large television instead of smaller computer monitor, would create the best picture, the "bigger is better" philosophy may not always be true for the videoconferencing images. Ultimately, even the best video camera may not display well if the screen (e.g., full-size monitor, laptop, tablet, smartphone) isn't optimal.

Desired Features

Display Screen Resolution and Size

To match a high-definition video camera, the provider should seek high-definition display screens that can provide 720p resolution or higher. As newer televisions, computer monitors, tablets, and smartphones are being released with higher-definition screens (e.g., 4K and higher possibilities), if one purchased such a product within the last few years, it is likely high definition, will complement the high-definition camera, and will suit the videoconferencing needs. However, if one is considering using an older display screen that is not high definition, or is considering pairing a high-definition display screen with a standard or lower-definition video camera, issues could arise. For example, lower-resolution video and a bigger display screen could increase the fuzziness of what is being displayed (Figure 8.1). In simplified terms, this is taking a video image that is meant to be a smaller resolution and thus size (i.e., less pixels) and attempting to stretch the image to fit a much larger screen than it was never designed to fit on. Unfortunately, as the video image is stretched to fit, new pixels aren't added to fill in the gaps in data, thus making the picture appear very blurry, which can have an observable negative impact on the video image. Think of this as trying to take a 2.5" x 3.5" wallet-sized photograph and stretching it onto a full-sized 20" x 24" painter's canvas. Everything would be stretched and look distorted, and thus, vastly inferior to the original. Contrastingly, having a high-resolution video image on a lower-resolution display screen can also decrease the quality of the image (Figure 8.2). In this situation, a larger video image that has a high resolution and thus larger size (i.e., more pixels), is attempting to be squished down to fit a smaller screen. In the attempt to make the higher-definition data fit the lower-resolution display screen, the image is being squeezed into a smaller size that it was never meant to be viewed in. Think of this as trying to take an advertisement on the size of a building and squeezing it down to a pocket-sized photo. In the squeezing, the data begins to compress, losing the clarity and detail of the images, and thus decreasing how it looks on the display screen.

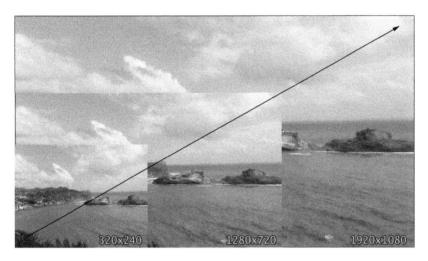

Figure 8.1 Low-resolution video image and larger display screen – increased fuzziness as the image is stretched to a larger display.

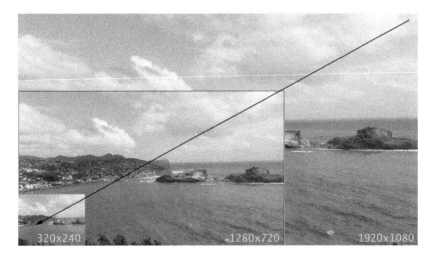

Figure 8.2 High-resolution video image and smaller display screens – decreased clarity and detail as the image is reduced to fit a smaller display.

Summary Points

- Display screens should have at least 720p video resolution for the video image, providers should seek complementing high-definition display screens.
- Displaying lower-resolution images on larger or high-definition display screens can stretch the image to a size not originally intended, creating distortion.
- Displaying higher-resolution images on a small or lower-definition display screens can squeeze the image to a size not originally intended, creating distortion.

9 Videoconferencing Logistics
Microphone Considerations

Complementing the video quality is audio quality. To capture the audio, an appropriate microphone is required. For many providers, a microphone built into a monitor, laptop, tablet, smartphone, or a plug-and-play USB camera can be an adequate way of capturing the verbal communication of both the provider and the patient. For providers requiring a clearer or more nuanced means of communicating, or if there is no adequate microphone available, a stand-alone dynamic of condenser microphone may be an option (Spargo et al., 2013). In such situations, the provider can either encourage the patient to purchase such a microphone, or loan one for the duration of the sessions.

Types of Microphones

Dynamic

Dynamic microphones (Figure 9.1) are some of the oldest designs (Wreglesworth, n.d.). Often used in music production due to their ability

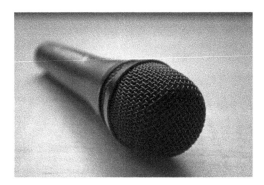

Figure 9.1 Example of dynamic microphone.

Source: Image from SennMicrophone.jpg (https://upload.wikimedia.org/wikipedia/commons/9/91/SennMicrophone.jpg) by ChrisEngelsma (July 28, 2009) (https://commons.wikimedia.org/w/index.php?title=User:ChrisEngelsma&action=edit&redlink=1) is licensed under CC BY-SA 3.0 (https://creativecommons.org/licenses/by-sa/3.0/deed.en).

to manage loud sounds and live instruments, dynamic microphones are useful in videoconferencing services due to being inexpensive, durable, and appropriate for general conversation-level discussions (Spargo et al., 2013; Wreglesworth, n.d.). Unfortunately, they are noted as not being very sensitive to quiet or higher-frequency sounds, meaning that if the provider or patient speaks more quietly, or is attempting more nuanced vocal expressions, they may not recognize such sounds well, requiring the users to pay closer attention to each other.

Condenser

Condenser microphones (Figure 9.2) are better suited for capturing quieter and more complex sounds than the dynamic microphones (Spargo et al., 2013; Wreglesworth, n.d.). These microphones are highly sensitive to sound and thus may be better suited for providers who require a microphone for either themselves or a patient that can capture not only quieter speech, but also a range of complex sounds (e.g., playing other videos or audio clips in session that need to be captured through the microphone for the patient, speaking softly as part of progressive muscle relaxation or an exposure technique). Contrasting with dynamic, condenser microphones are often more expensive, do not mange louder sounds as well, and are more delicate, requiring greater care (Spargo et al., 2013; Wreglesworth, n.d.).

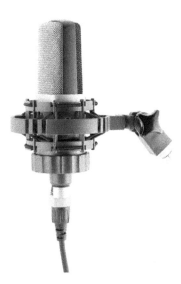

Figure 9.2 Example of condenser microphone.

Source: Image from AKG C214 Condenser Microphone with H85 Shock Mount. jpg (https://upload.wikimedia.org/wikipedia/commons/3/30/AKG_C214_condenser_microphone_with_H85_shock_mount.jpg) by Lucasbosch (March 28, 2014) (https://commons.wikimedia.org/wiki/User:Lucasbosch) is licensed under CC BY-SA 3.0 (https://creativecommons.org/licenses/by-sa/3.0/deed.en).

Desired Features

Easy to Install and Problem-Solve

As with any videoconferencing component, unless having a reasonable amount of technological knowledge, it is suggested that the provider and patient obtain microphones that are generally easy to install and problem-solve. If using a built-in microphone, little effort is required, and the microphone and software are likely already integrated. In this scenario, the provider and patient do not have to do anything else to make the microphone work with the videoconferencing platform. If one is to use a plug-and-play USB camera with built-in microphone, once the user plugs in the device, most computers will automatically configure it for immediate use with their system. However, if one is to seek out a separate dynamic or condenser microphone to supplement their video camera (i.e., using the camera only for video and turning off the microphone feature, microphone of camera does not work well or at all), they should ensure that the microphone suits their needs and can be easily used with their system. For example, while some are merely plug-and-play for immediate use, some higher-end microphones will install in a similar manner, but require calibration before it can be used in an effective way or without audio-related issues (e.g., feedback, picking up extraneous noises).

Summary Points

- Microphones can be built into the computer system the provider or patient is using (e.g., monitor, laptop, tablet, smartphone), built into a plug-and-play USB video camera and microphone combination, or be a standalone component.
- Microphones can be classified into two primary categories for videoconferencing use – dynamic and condenser.
- Dynamic microphones can be less costly, produce adequate sound, manage louder sounds more effectively, and be more durable to rough use.
- Condenser microphones can be more costly and less durable, but more sensitive to quieter and more complex sounds.
- The selected microphone should be easy to install, calibrate, and problem-solve.

References

Spargo, G., Karr, A., & Turvey, C. L. (2013). Technology options for the provision of mental health care through videoteleconferencing. In K. Myers & C. L. Turvey (Eds.), *Telemental health: Clinical, technical, and administrative foundations for evidence-based practice* (pp. 135–151). London: Elsevier.

Wreglesworth, R. (n.d.). What's the difference between dynamic and condenser microphones. *Musician's HQ.* Retrieved from https://musicianshq.com/whats-the-difference-between-dynamic-and-condenser-microphones/.

10 Videoconferencing Logistics

Videoconferencing Platform Considerations

Once a provider and patient have the proper equipment, one of the provider's biggest decisions is the selection of a videoconferencing platform. Over the last several years, the market has been flooded with companies claiming to be appropriate for videoconferencing psychotherapy and assessment, often with different marketing tactics to entice providers. Such variety can create challenges for knowing which platform may be best suited for a specific provider's practice. While there is no single "best" product, as what is best will likely vary by the unique demands of the provider, there are several specific considerations that should be evaluated to assist in selecting an appropriate platform. Given evolving needs, providers should consider selecting a platform that not only has functionality relevant to their current practice, but also has features that may become helpful in the future as the practice evolves based upon business or patient needs.

Primary Consideration Factors

Video and Audio Quality

To ensure clarity, the platform should allow for high-definition video and audio quality. Even the best video camera or microphone won't transmit the high-definition information if the videoconferencing platform limits the quality to a standard definition. As such, to support a high-definition video, the videoconferencing platform should support video resolution of at least 720p. Further, while high-definition may be desired, a videoconferencing platform with settings to modify the video and audio quality can be beneficial. For example, it is possible that either the provider or patient's internet may be limiting the connection and ability to smoothly transmit high-definition information at specific points in the sessions. As such, while telephone or another platform may be used, it may be possible to reduce the video quality from high definition to standard definition to stabilize the connection and continue the session on the original videoconferencing platform. While not as good as high definition, and likely not something the provider would like to do frequently, this approach could be viewed as superior to telephone in many ways, as users can still see and hear each other in real time.

General Functions

Supplementing video and audio quality are the general functions of the platform. These may include the aforementioned ability to increase or reduce the video quality, an ability to refresh the video or audio in real time to avoid having to "hang up" and reconnect, screen sharing (i.e., displaying what is on one user's screen to the other's), photo or video capture (i.e., recording or screenshot), an ability to "kick" disruptive users (e.g., for group therapy), and provider (i.e., host) settings to lock video and audio features for others. Additionally, some platforms have the option for virtual waiting rooms, with customization. Such "rooms" ensure that when patients connect to the platform (especially if they are early), they do not immediately and accidentally join an ongoing videoconferencing session of other patients. Rather, they are put into a queue, allowing the provider to select when they wish to allow the patient to enter the session. While some virtual waiting rooms (e.g., Doxy.me) are relatively simplistic, with the primary customization being the addition of a provider picture and changing of text (e.g., "Dr. _____ will be with you shortly"), others can be more complex. For instance, some waiting rooms (e.g., VSee Clinic) can have digital paperwork for patients to complete. Further, for providers who like more of a personal touch, some (e.g., Thera-Link) have options for differing imagery and music that can be used while patients wait for their session.

Number of Simultaneous Users

While potentially not a primary consideration for those who focus on individual therapy or commonly have only a small amount of video users in a single session (e.g., divorced family connected from two locations), for those conducting group therapy or who are seeing multiple people in different locations with different cameras, the number of simultaneous users allotted by the videoconferencing platform becomes very important. Platforms range in the number of allowed simultaneous users and can vary further by plan of the same platform. For example, some have limited user space, such as Doxy.me advertising ten simultaneous users (Doxy.me Help Center, n.d.). Alternatively, some platforms allow for substantially more, such as Zoom's paid versions. Zoom advertises plans allowing up to 100 video participants including the provider in a single meeting, with this number extended to 200–500 for large meeting plans (up to 100 panelists and 10,000 viewers for other plans; Zoom, 2015). Although a provider is unlikely to even require 30 simultaneous users in a single videoconferencing session, such numbers may be needed should a provider use the videoconferencing platform to conduct webinars or educational videoconferencing meetings, in addition to clinical matters. Ultimately, a provider should review the platforms of their choice to ensure that the number of users will match their practice and desired goals.

Security

The provider should take particular care in evaluating the videoconferencing platform's security features to ensure confidential transmission of information (Table 10.1). As further detailed in Chapter 4, the selected platform should include, at a minimum, password protection to restrict usage to only the intended users, and at least 128-bit encryption standards (NIST, 2001; Yellowlees et al., 2010). Detailing of security features is often readily available on a videoconferencing platform's website, or by contacting the company directly. Nevertheless, providers should do their homework, as some companies advertise "HIPAA compliance" on their website, but details of what this actually means or how they ensure the compliance are not always easily found, if they are listed at all. This is in contrast to many companies that readily provide their reported levels of encryption and security features, some of which may also include technical specifications for those interested in how the security actually works. For a

Table 10.1 Common videoconferencing platforms (2020)

Platforms that claim to meet HIPAA compliance standards*	*Platforms with questionable HIPAA compliance practices***
Adobe Connect	Facebook Messenger
Intermedia AnyMeeting	Facetime
BlueJeans	Google Hangouts (free)
Cisco WebEx	Skype (free)
ClockTree	Zoom (free)
Doxy.me	
Google G Suite	
GoToMeeting	
Microsoft Teams (replaced Skype for Business)	
Polycom	
SecureVideo	
Simple Practice	
Thera-Link	
Vidyo	
VSee	
Zoom for Healthcare	
Updox	

Notes: * Standards have been suggested to include at least 128-bit encryption, password protections, and will provide a signed BAA.

** Platforms may not detail their security or fail to provide a signed BAA.

provider, the more documented information, the better. Ultimately, it is the provider's responsibility to ensure the safety of the patient's e-PHI. When in doubt, it is suggested that the provider reach out to the videoconferencing platform and not only inquire about the security, but also request for the information in writing for their own documentation. If the information is available on their website, the provider can save the website information as a PDF, or take a screenshot for their records as well.

To ensure data protection and reduced liability of using the third-party videoconferencing platform, providers should seek a formalized and signed BAA outlining all pertinent aspects of the third-party's methods of storing and utilizing e-PHI (Baker & Stanley, 2018; HHS, 2013). While BAAs vary in detail provided, they should include an indication of adherence to the HIPAA Security Rule, as well as steps taken if breaches are recognized. Of note, while some companies have automated BAAs through their website, others require a provider to contact the platform's company to secure a signed BAA, potentially creating a gap from when the platform is purchased to when it can be used with a BAA in place. As such, the provider should question the amount of time required to receive a signed BAA prior to scheduling their videoconferencing sessions to ensure everything is in place prior to beginning or switching to the new method. It should be noted that it is a common practice for healthcare-focused videoconferencing platforms to offer BAAs. If a videoconferencing platform's company is unwilling to provide a BAA, the provider would be justified in being wary of their security standards.

Design

When selecting a videoconferencing platform, a provider should be aware that while some platforms were specifically designed for healthcare systems, others were not. For example, some have discussed the use of videoconferencing platforms that are often used for general meetings and business (e.g., Microsoft Teams, Cisco WebEx, GoToMeeting). Although potentially meeting the provider's needs, some may feel more comfortable securing a platform that markets itself as geared towards healthcare. If such a consideration is important to the provider, the platforms can be viewed as grouped into two primary categories. First are the standalone videoconferencing platforms that predominantly include the video program itself. These platforms (e.g., Doxy.me) have videoconferencing possibilities, as well as some customization settings including potential virtual waiting rooms. Alternatively, other platforms are full suites that include multiple components to ensure a streamlined workflow (e.g., VSee Clinic). Such components can include general functionality (e.g., waiting room, screen share, provider controls), as well as built in scheduling systems, hosting of online forms and educational information (e.g., articles, handouts), billing services, automated after-visit summaries, and scheduling reminders. Such higher-end services may also include live technical assistance if needed for either the provider or patient.

Integration with Current Systems

Depending on a provider's practice and use of other software beyond the videoconferencing platform, consideration may be given towards integration of the platform with preexisting programs. For example, some providers may already have EHR systems, such as the popular EPIC, that manage their documentation and scheduling. As such, while the provider may not require a full videoconferencing platform suite that would include redundant features, they may desire a videoconferencing platform that allows the video component to be seamlessly integrated with the preexisting EHR. Multiple companies have indicated the possibility of such integration, including Zoom and Vidyo (e.g., Barolo, 2020; VidyoHealth, n.d.). Integrating the videoconferencing into a preexisting EHR that contains the patient's medical record can not only be convenient, but can streamline the provider's workflow, allowing for all functions to be completed through a singular program as opposed to managing several.

Cost

Although potentially not the most important factor in a patient's direct care, cost can sometimes "make or break" a platform's potential for a provider. As a result of differing features and tiers of service, there are associated ranges of cost. Some platforms (e.g., Doxy.me, VSee) offer free basic videoconferencing services; however, these commonly lack key features, often offering only standard/lower-quality video, or not offering a BAA until one upgrades to paid versions. As such, while "free" can be enticing, it is often prudent for providers to purchase a full version to ensure the qualities desired and indicated for an ethical videoconferencing practice that meets HIPAA standards. Through a review of available platforms, providers will quickly recognize that they are predominantly subscription based, creating monthly or yearly charges, with cheaper monthly payments for longer subscriptions. Further complicating this is how some platforms have company or corporate versions that will allow for a set number of providers to use the platform for a designated price, while others charge per provider per month. As choosing can sometimes be difficult, it is suggested that the interested provider consult with peers who have used such platforms, as each contains both pros and cons. If a provider is unsure, some companies (e.g., ClockTree) offer free trial periods to test before deciding on continued payment. Finally, it should be noted that prices are ever-changing. As such, it would be wise for a provider to monitor for any fluctuations including from sales at key times of the year such as holidays and Black Friday. Just as entertainment products go on sale, so too do professional services.

Comparing Platforms

Given the multitude of companies advertising HIPAA-compliant video-conferencing platforms, combined with each company indicating differing features in terms of functionality, complexity, security, and costs, it can sometimes become challenging to consolidate the information to assist with a formal selection. As each provider must consider what is best for their practice, websites have created summary information pages to detail individual platforms, review platforms, and/or compare and contrast platforms (Table 10.2).

Table 10.2 Websites to assist in the selection of a videoconferencing platform

Name	Weblink
Person Centered Tech	https://personcenteredtech.com/pct_vendorreview_tag/videoconferencing/
Telebehavioral Health Institute	https://telehealth.org/telehealth-buyers-guide/wpbdp_category/videoconferencing/
Telemental Health Comparisons	https://telementalhealthcomparisons.com/

Summary Points

- When determining an appropriate videoconferencing platform, providers should consider the video and audio quality, general functions (e.g., real-time refreshing of quality, screen sharing, photo or video capture, the ability to "kick" disruptive users, virtual waiting rooms), allotted number of simultaneous users, platform security (e.g., passwords, encryption standards, signed BAA), intended design and integration with other provider systems, and costs.
- Providers should consider a videoconferencing platform that not only suits their current needs, but one that has additional features that may be helpful as one's practice evolves as based upon either business or patient needs.

References

Baker, J., & Stanley, A. (2018). Telemedicine technology: A review of services, equipment, and other aspects. *Current Allergy and Asthma Reports*, *18*(11), 60. https://doi.org/10.1007/s11882-018-0814-6.

Barolo, P. (2020, April 7). Introducing Zoom for telehealth. Zoom Blog. Retrieved from https://blog.zoom.us/wordpress/2017/04/20/introducing-zoom-for-tele health/.

Doxy.me Help Center. (n.d.). Group call: Add multiple participants to a call. Doxy.me. Retrieved from https://help.doxy.me/en/articles/95902-group-call-add-multiple-participants-to-a-call.

National Institute of Standards and Technology (NIST). (2001). *Federal Information Processing Standards Publication 197: Announcing the advanced encryption standard (AES)*. Retrieved from https://nvlpubs.nist.gov/nistpubs/FIPS/NIST.FIPS.197.pdf.

US Health and Human Services (HHS). (2013). *Business associate contracts.* Retrieved from www.hhs.gov/hipaa/for-professionals/covered-entities/sample-business-associate-agreement-provisions/index.html.

VidyoHealth. (n.d.). VidyoHealth. Retrieved from www.vidyo.com/video-conferencing-solutions/industry/telehealth.

Yellowlees, P., Shore, J., & Roberts, L. (2010). Practice guidelines for videoconferencing telemental health, October 2009. *Telemedicine Journal and e-Health, 16*(10), 1074–1089. https://doi.org/10.1089/tmj.2010.0148.

Zoom. (2015, May 27). Top 3 zoomer Q & A. Retrieved from https://blog.zoom.us/wordpress/2015/05/27/top-3-zoomer-q-a/.

11 Videoconferencing Logistics
Bandwidth and Latency Considerations

Although high-speed internet has become commonplace throughout a large portion of the United States, a provider should be aware of the influences of both bandwidth and latency on the video and audio quality of the videoconferencing sessions. While often used interchangeably, there are differences in the two constructs. Nevertheless, both are equally important considerations.

Bandwidth

Bandwidth refers to the maximum rate of data transfer per second over an internet connection (Glueck, 2013; Prasad et al., 2003; Tuerk et al., 2015). It is most often measured in bits per second (BPS; Spargo et al., 2013). More specifically, the rate can vary between 1,000 bits per second (i.e., kilobits per second, KBPS), 1,000,000 bits per second (i.e., megabits per second, MBPS), or 1,000,000,000 bits per second (i.e., gigabits per second, GBPS). In videoconferencing terms, KBPS produces low quality, MBPS produces good quality, and GBPS produces the best quality. While there are limited discussions of appropriate bandwidth for videoconferencing, the ATA's *Practice Guidelines for Videoconferencing Telemental Health* (Yellowlees et al., 2010) suggested the use of 384 KBPS or higher transmission to ensure the smooth and natural communication pace for video encounters. For simple one-to-one video calling, 384 KBPS may be sufficient, however, for higher definitions and more users, higher bandwidth would likely be required.

Latency

Latency refers to the time required for a signal to travel from a source to a destination (Armstrong & Dilley, 2020; Schafer, 2019). In simple terms, this is the delay of how long it takes data to travel from one point to another, often measured in milliseconds by round-trip time (RTT; Spero, n.d.). For example, low latency for a high-speed internet connection makes online pages load almost immediately. As such, low latency is good for videoconferencing, as it means there is little to no lag, while high latency can create difficulties. Although no detailing by guiding organizations are available related to latency, some technical outlets have suggested ≤ 150 milliseconds of one-way latency from mouth to ear for videoconferencing. As indicated by technical outlets, delays of approximately 200 milliseconds are human-perceptible and can create issues (Poly, 2019). For more tech-savvy readers, the 150 millisecond benchmark includes ≤ 30 milliseconds of jitter (i.e., inconsistency in the latency of packets with lower numbers being more desirable) and ≤ 1 percent packet loss (i.e., discarded or lost packet information with lower numbers being more desirable; Campbell, 2011; Lewis & Pickavance, 2006; Poly, 2019).

Testing Speeds

As bandwidth and latency are more technical discussions, providers may be unsure of how to evaluate such constructs. Two helpful resources that test several aspects of a user's videoconferencing components include WebRTC Troubleshooter (https://test.webrtc.org) and Vonage's Pre-Call Test (https://tokbox.com/developer/tools/precall/). These tools check the connectivity, media access, and quality of both video and audio connections. More specifically for videoconferencing, the tests determine if the user's network will support different video qualities, including high-definition video. As part of this analysis, bandwidth and latency are reported. Of note, Vonage's Pre-Call Test provides a bitrate stability measure to estimate the expected videoconferencing call quality for both video and audio, independently.

Once a session begins, especially as it relates to psychological and neuropsychological assessment procedures, providers may want to have latency checks to ensure that responses are immediate and not delayed. Some of the easiest ways to accomplish this are "low tech" and involve engaging the patient in a series of tasks to see how long it takes them to react. For example, to test the video latency, the provider could ask that the patient raise their index finger on the count of three. If there is low latency, the actions should be relatively immediate and smooth. If it takes the patient several additional seconds to raise their finger on the provider's screen, then lag is likely present. If lag presents, the degree can be estimated, and equipment can be evaluated and adjusted, if possible. A similar process can be used for audio integrity. In this scenario, the provider counts down to three for the patient to say a specific word or phrase. Video and audio checks can also be reversed with the patient testing the provider's latency. Of significant note, it should be emphasized that such methods are intended for individuals who do not exhibit cognitive or physical slowing, as their slowing could be perceived as a latency issue if not accounted for by the provider.

Summary Points

- Bandwidth and latency are two important constructs for videoconferencing processes.
- The ATA recommends a bandwidth of at least 384 KBPS for therapeutic videoconferencing, but higher amounts may be required for higher definitions or more users.
- A latency of ≤ 150 milliseconds with ≤ 30 milliseconds of jitter and ≤ 1 percent packet loss can be considered optimal for videoconferencing.
- Online tools can help a provider or patient evaluate the bandwidth and latency.
- Latency checks can be used throughout the processes to ensure video and audio integrity.

References

Armstrong, R. L., & Dilley, J. (2020, March 25). The consumer's guide to Internet speed. HighSpeedInternet.com. Retrieved from www.highspeedinternet.com/resources/the-consumers-guide-to-internet-speed#bandwidth.

Campbell, S. (2011, December). Video conferencing bandwidth requirements for the WAN. *TechTarget*. Retrieved from https://searchnetworking.techtarget.com/tip/Video-conferencing-bandwidth-requirements-for-the-WAN#:~:text=Target%20values%20for%20acceptable%20video, parameter%20somewhat%20difficult%20to%20control.

Glueck, D. (2013). Establishing therapeutic rapport in telemental health. In K. Myers & C. L. Turvey (Eds.), *Telemental health: Clinical, technical, and administrative foundations for evidence-based practice* (pp. 29–46). London: Elsevier.

Lewis, C., & Pickavance, S. (2006, May 26). Implementing quality of service over Cisco MPLS VPNs. *Cisco*. Retrieved from www.ciscopress.com/articles/article.asp?p=471096&seqNum=6.

Poly. (2019). *Preparing your IP network for video conferencing: And workarounds for less than ideal conditions*. Retrieved from https://support.polycom.com/content/dam/polycom-support/products/uc-infrastructure-support/management-scheduling/dma/other-documents/en/preparing-ip-network-video-conferencing.pdf.

Prasad, R., Dovrolis, C., Murray, M., & Claffy, K. C. (2003). Bandwidth estimation: Metrics, measurement techniques, and tools. *IEEE Network, 17*(6), 27–35. https://doi.org/10.1109/MNET.2003.1248658.

Schafer, D. (2019, December 23). Bandwidth vs. latency: What is the difference? HighSpeedInternet.com. Retrieved from www.highspeedinternet.com/resources/bandwidth-vs-latency-what-is-the-difference.

Spargo, G., Karr, A., & Turvey, C. L. (2013). Technology options for the provision of mental health care through videoteleconferencing. In K. Myers & C. L. Turvey (Eds.), *Telemental health: Clinical, technical, and administrative foundations for evidence-based practice* (pp. 135–151). London: Elsevier.

Spero, S. E. (n.d.). Analysis of HTTP performance problems. *W3C*. Retrieved from www.w3.org/Protocols/HTTP-NG/http-prob.html.

Tuerk, P. W., Ronzio, J. L., & Shore, P. (2015). Technologies and clinical video-conferencing infrastructures: A guide to selecting appropriate systems. In P. W. Tuerk & P. Shore (Eds.), *Clinical videoconferencing in telehealth: Program development and practice* (pp. 3–22). Cham: Springer International.

Yellowlees, P., Shore, J., & Roberts, L. (2010). Practice guidelines for videoconferencing telemental health, October 2009. *Telemedicine and e-Health, 16*(10), 1074–1089. https://doi.org/10.1089/tmj.2010.0148.

12 Videoconferencing Logistics
Room Setup Considerations

In order to maximize the videoconferencing, the provider should consider how the rooms are set up at both the provider and patient's locations. An appropriate setup can foster positive attitudes and experiences, while a provider failing to appropriately consider and address issues can create a range of negative perceptions, leading to challenges that could impede the therapeutic activities (Simpson et al., 2016). Broadly defined, room setup considerations can include the room size, general room selection and background appearance, privacy and interruptions, lighting, and camera placement.

Room Size

While perhaps not as important of a consideration for the provider who is independently in an office setting, the size of the room can significantly impact the patient's therapeutic services (Goldstein & Glueck, 2016; Luxton et al., 2016, chap. 6; Maheu et al., 2001). When care is provided in a distant clinical location, such as in a patient's home, the provider should coach the patient in the selection of a room that is not only conducive to the therapeutic services, but allows the provider to observe all members in the room. For example, if a provider is to meet with a patient who remains seated in front of a camera, a larger space may not be needed for most sessions. However, if a provider will want the patient to move, use available objects for practice exercises, or interact with additional members in the room (e.g., couples or family therapy), a larger space will be required. Further, more space may be helpful for those individuals who have trouble siting for extended periods of time, such as those with attention difficulties, or physical discomfort from not moving for extended periods. Ultimately, the room should be large enough that the patient can sit, stand, and move comfortably, although some adjustment of the camera may be necessary for a moving patient. While adults may not require significant space if met with independently, providers should consider if children will be present, either as part of the treatment, or due to requiring supervision. For children, especially if they are patients, the space should allow for the caregivers to comfortably sit, while also allowing space for the children to play without bumping into each other or other objects, all while remaining in the camera's view (Goldstein & Glueck, 2016; Luxton et al., 2016, chap. 6; Myers et al., 2017). Of note, a provider should also avoid too large or over decorated rooms for themselves or the patients, as such rooms can create distractions for either an adult or child (Yellowlees et al., 2010). Further, too large of a room may allow patients to move out of the frame of the camera during therapeutic activities.

General Room Selection and Background Appearance

While not always achievable, ideally, both the provider's and patient's room should appear as close as possible to a normal office or consulting room. This can help foster attitudes that the videoconferencing processes are healthcare practices and should not be diminished merely because it is outside of the normal office settings. Unfortunately, some have chronicled how negative attitudes towards videoconferencing can be influenced by the environment itself, removed from the actual quality of the interactions between the provider and patient (Simpson et al., 2016). For the provider, the appearance and decorations should be relatively plain, clean, and uncluttered in order to create a pleasant ambiance. Further, one should avoid dark backgrounds, as this can create a strong contrast with the lighted images (Maheu et al., 2001). Alternatively, as summarized by Jones and colleagues (2006), some have suggested the use of midrange blue backgrounds, which have been suggested to facilitate better quality for many skin tones. The goal is to furnish the office as one would in person to create a welcoming and professional atmosphere (Luxton et al., 2016, chap. 6). Special consideration should be given to what is behind the provider in the video image's view. This means that providers should strive to have a clear and clean background, without paperwork or books all over their desks or behind them. Further, providers should avoid having a backdrop of a bookshelf, or other "busy" furniture or artwork (Luxton et al., 2016, chap. 6; Simpson et al., 2016). While some may think that backdrops of books or papers on a desk can make the provider appear more professional, consider that the objects could be distracting, not only for the average person, but potentially more so for a patient with a diagnosed history of attention-deficit/hyperactivity disorder (ADHD), OCD, or another diagnosis that may lead to a focus on the distractions (e.g., thoughts about clutter, someone trying to read the book titles, noticing that books or papers are not evenly aligned). For providers who are unable to find an optimal location or rearrange an office, an alternative is to merely block the background. The simplest means of accomplishing this is through background blocking devices. For example, some have used a portable room divider (Figure 12.1), sometimes referred to as folding screens or privacy screens, that can be set up behind the provider to block all other viewable space. Similarly, one can use a portable webcam background screen that can be attached to the back of an office chair, such as Webaround's "The Big Shot" (Figure 12.2). These portable screens can be used to block backgrounds, and are also often solid blue or green to allow for chroma keying in which one can replace the blue or green color with another background image for fun video calls with child patients, or with the provider's friends and family.

As best as possible, similar recommendations should be applied to the patient's location. To accomplish this, providers can coach the patient in cleaning up or rearranging a specific area or room to become the "therapy room." As patients may present in a wide range of locations, this can sometimes be challenging. For example, some patients may present from a distant clinic that already has an acceptable preset layout. Others may have a single or multi-bedroom apartment or condominium that may have limited rooms, requiring modification of the available space. Further, while some may have a house with many room options, merely having a large amount of space is only part of the challenge, as even the largest of spaces may not be conducive to videoconferencing if they are overly cluttered, or are occupied by people who are not participating in the therapeutic processes. As such, providers may sometimes have to "get creative" and collaborate with the patient to create a location for the videoconferencing. Unfortunately, sometimes real-life situations do not allow for an appropriate room. While not ideal, some providers have reported having videoconferencing sessions while the patient is alone in their car or a bathroom due to no other locations, inside or out of the home, being available.

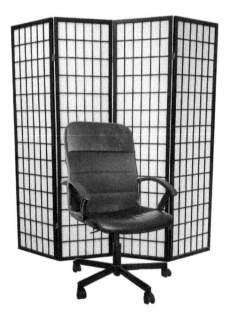

Figure 12.1 Example of generic foldable screen.

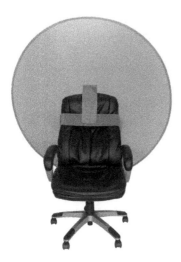

Figure 12.2 Example background screen – Webaround's "The Big Shot" foldable webcam backdrop.

Source: Image copyrighted 2019 by Bobachi, LLC, and included with permission (Webaround, n.d; https://thewebaround.com/product/the-big-shot/).

Privacy and Interruptions

To ensure privacy and confidentiality, a provider and patient should select rooms that can allow for an appropriate speech volume without letting people outside of the room hear or see them. More specifically, the room should be one with shut doors, both covered and closed windows, and thicker walls. In supplement of these factors, the space should limit interruptions (Luxton et al., 2016, chap. 6; Luxton et al., 2014). With consideration of safety of both the patient and others, door locks may be helpful to limit others disturbing the sessions. This may be especially helpful if other members of the location, including children, are prone to coming in and out of the room during the videoconferencing sessions.

In addition to the physical safeguards, the provider and patients can minimize interruptions by explaining to others that the sessions are important, and they should avoid interrupting unless for specific reasons, such as emergencies. To indicate that sessions are occurring, both the provider and patient may wish to have a physical indication, such as a sign saying, "Please Do Not Disturb." While a general door sign may be sufficient, people can become more creative, including the use of a countdown clock, humorous signs that can be created in collaboration with an interrupting child, or the use of lights (e.g., holiday lights; Figures 12.3 and 12.4).

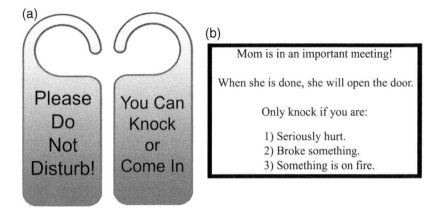

Figure 12.3 Examples of "Do Not Disturb" signs for a patient's home.

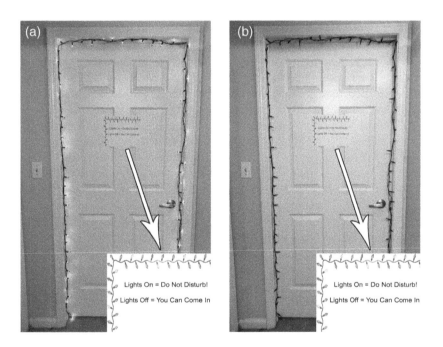

Figure 12.4 Examples of "Do Not Disturb" lights for a patient's home.

To further increase privacy and reduce outside interruptions, a provider should advise the patient to silence their phones and other interrupting items at the onset of each session. Similarly, the provider should advise the patient to unplug voice-activated devices such as Amazon Alexa, Echo Dots, Google Home, and Apple HomePod that can accidentally activate or collect information (Day et al., 2019; Needleman & Olson, 2019; O'Flaherty, 2019). Finally, should a patient (or provider) be struggling with outside noise limiting their focus, they can consider the use of noise-cancelling headphones. Alternatively, white noise machines can be placed at the doorway to decrease outside noise, and increase privacy (Goldstein & Glueck, 2016).

Lighting

To ensure that both the provider and patient are able to be clearly seen in the video image, the provider should consider the lighting at both locations (Krupinski & Leistner, 2017). In part, this process involves the evaluation of whether to use natural versus artificial lighting, or both. More specifically, while natural light through a nearby window can be helpful at illuminating the user, too much direct light can result in washed-out images. To control for this, the provider or patient can consider the use of blinds or shades, as well as artificial lighting. If using artificial, the provider should emphasize the use of warm and diffuse colors, ideally yellows, while avoiding use of more distorting colors, such as bright reds or oranges, violets, blues, and greens (Krupinski & Leistner, 2017; Luxton et al., 2016, chap. 6; Simpson et al., 2016). When it comes to the specific type of artificial light to use or avoid, disagreements have occurred in the literature. While some have suggested that providers avoid fluorescent lighting (e.g., Simpson et al., 2016), others have indicated that warm fluorescents can be an acceptable choice (e.g., Krupinski & Leistner, 2017; Luxton et al., 2016, chap. 6). It is up to the provider to test the options to determine what is best for their needs. Ultimately, for some, the selection may simply come down to what is available.

With the lighting type selected, the provider should set up their own room, and coach the patient in ways to maximize even lighting to create the best video image possible. Unfortunately, poor lighting can lead to images that are distorted, and can also reduce the ability to see nuanced behaviors (e.g., facial expression changes). Further, poor lighting can create unflattering dark facial shadows, including under one's eyes (Krupinski & Leistner, 2017; Maheu et al., 2001). To correct for this, primary lighting should be behind the camera and aimed directly onto the provider or patient (Luxton et al., 2016, chap. 6; Maheu et al., 2001). If the primary source is overhead, but is insufficient or causing image issues, a provider or patient can use a standing lamp, small light clamp that can be put onto a computer monitor or tablet, or another light source to compensate (Luxton et al., 2016, chap. 6).

Camera Placements

Angles for Image Quality

Complementing the lighting, the camera placements and angles can create a clear or distorted image quality. The camera should be positioned in a way that avoids silhouetting (Figure 12.5), which can occur when there is too much backlighting from a window or light, making the person shadowed and difficult to see (Angus, 2020; Krupinski & Leistner, 2017; Simpson et al., 2016). Further, providers and patients should avoid placing the camera with hallways, windows, mirrors, or reflective materials behind them, as each can create distractions and potential difficulties for the image due to reflections or background motion (Angus, 2020; Simpson et al., 2016). Further, if a doorway is behind the provider or patient, it may be helpful to place a towel or other blocking material by the base to reduce shadows of others walking by. This may be especially important if the provider or patient has multiple people who may be walking by the room, or if they have pets that may be pacing or attempting to sniff under the door.

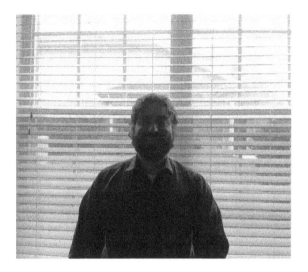

Figure 12.5 Example of silhouetting from background lighting.

Angles to Include All Participants

If working with a single patient who generally remains seated, the camera angle may not be a large consideration. However, if multiple adults are sitting next to each other, new members will be joining the session, or if children are sitting on the floor in addition to caregivers sitting on a chair or couch, the provider must consider the optimal angle to ensure everyone is in the view. If a provider has access to a camera at the patient's location that allows for zooming, tilting, and panning, such features can be used to adjust the camera in real time. If such features are not available, the provider can coach the patient to rearrange the camera to capture a broader view. For example, the camera can be pushed back to capture a wider angle (Myers et al., 2017). While this approach may be the simplest and allow for a better view of everyone in the room, it also creates new issues. Most importantly, moving a camera back may reduce the provider's ability to see more nuanced and smaller behaviors of those in the videoconferencing session. Ultimately, it is the provider's judgment as to what angles will be best for the therapeutic processes, with some choices being functional as based upon available options, but not optimal.

Angles for Eye Gaze

Beyond image quality, camera placement associated with eye contact is important for therapeutic rapport. This telepresence, or eye-gaze angle, is the angle between the eye and the camera, and the eye and the center of the display screen (Goldstein & Glueck, 2016; Luxton et al., 2014; Tam et al., 2007). In a practical sense, this process involves placement of the patient's image so that their head and eyes are in close proximity to the provider's video camera. In doing so, by looking at the video image, it appears as though the provider is looking into the camera and thus making direct eye contact with the patient. For example, if the image of the patient and the camera are not well aligned (e.g., the image of the patient is on the bottom of the screen, while the camera is on the top of the monitor), the provider may be looking at the image of the patient on their screen, but appearing on the patient's screen as looking down rather than "at them." Unfortunately, this can present as the provider appearing disengaged (Figure 12.6). As such, the provider should strive to create camera-viewing angles that appear as close to a normal conversation as possible. While setups will vary, if the camera is at the top of the display screen, the patient should be positioned to have their head and eyes close to the top of the screen (i.e., closest to the camera). Alternatively, a detachable camera can be moved to another location to match the video image of the patient. If the camera is built into the computer (i.e., cannot be moved), such as those in laptops, and placing the laptop on a regular desk makes the provider appear as

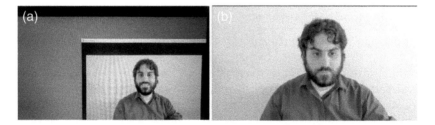

Figure 12.6 Example of the importance of camera alignment to simulate eye contact: (a) patient's image is placed on the bottom right of the provider's display screen away from a top-centered camera; (b) how the provider presents to the patient due to the provider having to look at the bottom right of their screen.

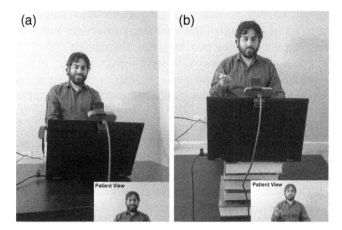

Figure 12.7 Example of raising a laptop to create a more natural eye gaze: (a) laptop placed significantly below eye level, resulting in downward eye gaze to patient; (b) laptop raised on books to ensure camera is eye level, resulting in natural eye gaze to patient.

though they are looking down at the patient due to the angle of the laptop (i.e., the screen and camera must be angled up due to being so low on the table), the provider can use books or other materials to raise the laptop to direct eye contact height (Figure 12.7). While computers and laptops are considered by many to be the optimal means of videoconferencing, some patients may only have access to a tablet or smartphone. Although such patients can attempt to angle the tablet or smartphone against an object or a wall, they could also utilize a desk or wall bracket, or a cellphone/tablet stand to hold the device at an appropriate height and angle.

Of important note, although eye contact is an important consideration, it should be viewed within the context of a patient's cultural factors. For example, the ATA (Ben-Arieh et al., 2016) has summarized that in relation to telehealth services, Arabs, Latin Americans, and Southern Europeans make more eye contact during conversation than Asians and Northern Europeans, while Japanese individuals specifically may consider eye contact rude. Due to this, beyond general angles, the provider should consider the potential impact that their eye contact has on the videoconferencing in a similar way that they would with F2F interactions. As with F2F methods, clarifying the patient's values and expectations, as well as their desire for increased or decreased eye contact may be helpful at the onset of services in order to avoid any misunderstandings.

Use of Two Cameras for Multi-Views

For providers who may require different views of a single room, multiple cameras can be utilized. Multiple cameras may become helpful should a provider have more than one patient in a room that may need to be viewed simultaneously, but cannot fit into a single camera view. Additionally, the administration and scoring of psychological or neuropsychological assessments may require that the provider view the patient's larger body (e.g., torso and up) to make behavioral observations, while also observing their hands to monitor manipulatives, view written or drawing activities, and to establish the patient's processes and time required for completion of tasks.

Setting up two cameras can be done in multiple ways. While tech-savvy providers can consider the use of USB video mixers, for those not familiar with this more complex method, they can opt for one of two simpler solutions. The first way to implement two cameras is to use a video-conferencing platform that has such features already built in. In doing so, the provider, patient, or provider's representative at the patient's location would need to appropriately set up the two cameras as the patient's site. As an example, one of the cameras can be built into the computer system (e.g., laptop built-in camera), while another is a plug-and-play USB camera. Alternatively, two plug-and-play USB cameras can be used (Figure 12.8). Once the cameras are set up and angled to the provider's specifications, they can be viewed. While not all platforms allow for such functionality, some have a specific setting for use of two cameras. Using Zoom as an example, the users start by beginning a normal videoconferencing session. The patient or representative who is setting up the session can then be coached by the distant provider to select the "share a second screen" option. Of note, the provider (i.e., host) may need to provide access for the patient to utilize such features. Among the options for sharing a second screen is the ability to share a second camera. While some rearrangement of the multiple views

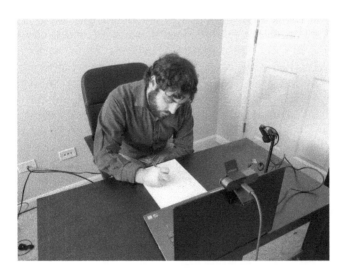

Figure 12.8 Use of two independent cameras with a single computer system.

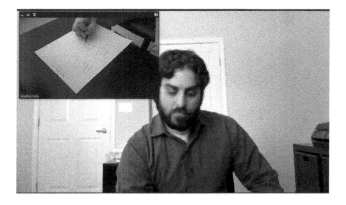

Figure 12.9 Example of provider's screen when using second-camera screen share in Zoom.

may be required for the provider's screen, this should allow the provider to see the two cameras simultaneously (Figure 12.9). As different platforms and computer systems (e.g., differing amounts of USB ports available to plug in additional cameras) vary in their ability to manage two cameras simultaneously, the provider should "do their homework" when considering a videoconferencing platform, if it is an important feature for them.

A second way requires additional equipment, but is more applicable to a wider range of videoconferencing platforms. This method requires two systems (e.g., desktop computer and laptop, laptop and laptop, laptop and tablet) and two separate cameras (e.g., built-in, plug-and-play USB) at the patient's location. In essence, the provider would create the initial videoconferencing session as normal to connect the provider and patient. The patient or provider's representative at the patient's site would then add the second patient's computer system and camera as a third caller to the already running videoconferencing session. Using Doxy.me as an example, the provider can add a "second caller" as a group call. Instead of having three separate callers, the patient is sharing two unique views of the single location (i.e., as two of the caller windows). In this method, one system and camera are set up on the primary viewing angle of the patient, likely the torso and up to view the individual and foster an appropriate eye-gaze angle. The second system and camera would be set up and angled to capture the secondary desired location, including a view of the patient's hands during assessment procedures (Figure 12.10).

Special Considerations for Young Children Using Toys in the Session Room

When working with children and preparing a room for F2F sessions, it is often wise to have a small selection of toys available for play (Myers et al.,

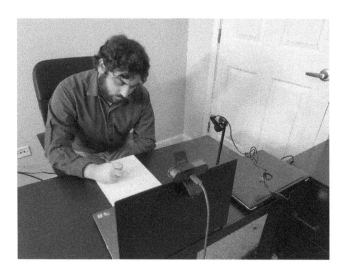

Figure 12.10 Example of using two independent laptop computers and two independent cameras.

2017). This approach should also be employed for videoconferencing. While desirable for a variety of reasons (e.g., to observe behavior and frustration tolerance, observe fine motor control, observe attention level), toys should be selected to foster a successful session, and as such, families will likely require guidance from the provider on acceptable types. With consideration of what is required for the child's treatment (e.g., if specific kinds of toys are required for parent–child interaction therapy), the provider should coach the family to encourage toys that are not noisy, multicomponent, messy, or require frequent redirection to avoid the child hurting themselves or another (Myers et al., 2017). Cars, trains, planes, dolls, figures, crayons for coloring, and simple connector sets may all be reasonable. Toys that make noise, encourage banging or destruction (e.g., tools), and those that will require substantial cleanup at the end of the session may want to be avoided. While these guidelines are generally acceptable to caregivers and children, some may ask, "what about Lego?" The use of Lego bricks and other building blocks will likely depend on the child themselves. If the child is able to play quietly, the blocks may be okay. However, for children who frequently dig for specific block types, or like to noisily dump all the pieces on the floor before putting them back into the box over and over, Lego bricks and other blocks may be reserved for outside of the videoconferencing sessions. Although the noise may not seem like a lot to the caregivers and child, the noise can be amplified through the microphone, making it difficult for the provider to hear what the patient or family are saying (Myers et al., 2017).

Summary Points

- The provider should consider the size of the videoconferencing room. For the patient, the room should be large enough so that they can freely move and stand, while remaining in the video camera's frame. This may be especially important for children, who may need to move around on the floor. Nevertheless, one does not want a room so large that the patient can leave the frame.
- The room's appearance has been suggested to influence the patient's attitudes towards the videoconferencing process, as well as therapeutic rapport. The provider should use and encourage rooms that mirror a normal office to maintain the professionalism of the therapeutic processes. The appearance should ideally be relatively plain, clean, uncluttered, and devoid of distracting background materials in order to create a pleasant ambiance. Background blocking devices can be used for busier settings that cannot be easily rearranged or modified.
- The provider should encourage privacy and minimal interruptions for all locations. Ensuring privacy should include selecting rooms that reduce the ability for nondesired individuals to see into. The selected room should also not allow those outside of it to hear what is being discussed. "Do Not Disturb" signs or other creative means of reducing distractions, while simple, can be very helpful, especially for children prone to interrupting. Noise machines may also be helpful for increasing privacy.
- Providers should encourage proper lighting at both their and their patient's locations to ensure appropriate image quality. Specifically, all members should create even lighting, while reducing shadows or silhouetting.
- Providers should ensure proper camera angles at both the provider's and the patient's locations. Angles can assist with general image quality, as well as reducing distractions (e.g., avoiding pointing towards hallways, windows, mirrors, reflective materials). Angles can also foster telepresence, also referred to as eye-gaze angle, which can assist in establishing and maintaining therapeutic rapport.
- Two cameras can sometimes be used, varying by available equipment. Two cameras can be helpful for larger spaces that may include multiple people, or for assessment procedures that require views of both the larger view of the person, as well as a focus on their hands to view manipulatives or written procedures to evaluate the patient's processes and time required for completion.
- If involving children, the provider should coach the family in selecting appropriate toys that will not be disruptive to the session.

References

Angus, T. (2020, April 1). Looking better on video calls. *Imperial Photography Digest*. Retrieved from wwwf.imperial.ac.uk/blog/photography/2020/04/01/looking-better-on-video-calls/.

Ben-Arieh, D., Charness, N., Duckett, K., Krupinski, E., Leistner, G., & Strawderman, L. (2016). *A concise guide for telemedicine practitioners: Human factors quick guide eye contact.* Arlington, VA: American Telemedicine Association. Retrieved from www.americantelemed.org/resources/a-concise-guide-for-telemedicine-practitioners-human-factors-quick-guide-eye-contact/.

Day, M., Turner, G., & Drozdiak, N. (2019, April 10). Amazon workers are listening to what you tell Alexa. *Bloomberg*. Retrieved from www.bloomberg.com/news/articles/2019-04-10/is-anyone-listening-to-you-on-alexa-a-global-team-reviews-audio.

Goldstein, F., & Glueck, D. (2016). Developing rapport and therapeutic alliance during telemental health sessions with children and adolescents. *Journal of Child and Adolescent Psychopharmacology, 26*(3), 204–211. https://doi.org/10.1089/cap.2015.0022.

Jones, R. M., Leonard, S., & Birmingham, L. (2006). Setting up a telepsychiatry service. Psychiatric Bulletin, 30(12), 464–467. https://doi.org/10.1192/pb.30.12.464.

Krupinski, E., & Leistner, G. (2017). *Let there be light: A quick guide to telemedicine lighting.* Arlington, VA: American Telemedicine Association. Retrieved from www.americantelemed.org/resources/let-there-be-light-a-quick-guide-to-telemedicine-lighting/.

Luxton, D. D., Nelson, E. -L., & Maheu, M. M. (2016). *A practitioner's guide to telemental health: How to conduct legal, ethical, and evidence-based telepractice.* Washington, DC: American Psychological Association.

Luxton, D. D., Pruitt, L. D., & Osenbach, J. E. (2014). Best practices for remote psychological assessment via telehealth technologies. *Professional Psychology: Research and Practice, 45*(1), 27–35. https://doi.org/10.1037/a0034547.

Maheu, M. M., Whitten, P., & Allen, A. (2001). Appendix C: Videoconferencing room requirements and etiquette. In M. M. Maheu, P. Whitten, & A. Allen (Eds.), *e-Health, telehealth, and telemedicine: A guide to start-up and success* (pp. 307–313). San Francisco, CA: Jossey-Bass.

Myers, K., Nelson, E. -L., Rabinowitz, T., Hilty, D., Baker, D., Barnwell, S. S., … Bernard, J. (2017). American Telemedicine Association practice guidelines for telemental health with children and adolescents. *Telemedicine and e-Health, 23*(10), 779–804. https://doi.org/10.1089/tmj.2017.0177.

Needleman, S. E., & Olson, P. (2019, July 11). Google contractors listen to recordings of people using virtual assistant. *Wall Street Journal*. Retrieved from www.wsj.com/articles/google-contractors-listen-to-recordings-of-consumers-addressing-virtual-assistant-11562865883.

O'Flaherty, K. (2019, April 12). Amazon staff are listening to Alexa conversations – Here's what to do. *Forbes*. Retrieved from www.forbes.com/sites/kateoflahertyuk/2019/04/12/amazon-staff-are-listening-to-alexa-conversations-heres-what-to-do/#adf8a3a71a22.

Simpson, S., Richardson, L., & Reid, C. (2016). Therapeutic alliance in videoconferencing psychotherapy. In S. Goss, K. Anthony, L. S. Stretch, & D. M. Nagel (Eds.), *Technology in mental health: Applications in practice, supervision, and training* (2nd ed., pp. 99–116). Springfield, IL: Charles C. Thomas.

Tam, T., Cafazzo, J. A., Seto, E., Salenieks, M. E., & Rossos, P. G. (2007). Perception of eye contact in video teleconsultation. *Journal of Telemedicine and Telecare, 13*(1), 35–39. https://doi.org/10.1258/135763307779701239.

Yellowlees, P., Shore, J., & Roberts, L. (2010). Practice guidelines for videoconferencing telemental health, October 2009. *Telemedicine and e-Health, 16*(10), 1074–1089. https://doi.org/10.1089/tmj.2010.0148.

13 Videoconferencing Logistics
Video Tips

As a provider prepares to begin a videoconferencing assessment or treatment session, steps should be taken to ensure the clarity and quality of the video image (Luxton et al., 2014; Myers et al., 2017). A clear video image can facilitate rapport, as well as the collection of information through direct and real-time behavioral observations. As it can sometimes be difficult for a provider or patient to recognize how they appear on another person's videoconferencing screen, the provider should take steps to maximize their own video image, and also to guide the patient. The following are tips to foster proper video image throughout the sessions. Tips can be broadly classified as relating to clothing, before-session factors, during-session factors, and post-session factors.

Clothing

While people often wish to "look good" for videoconferencing, careful consideration should be given to the type of clothing one wears. More specifically, providers and patients should avoid highly textured, striped, checkered, or patterned clothing. Further, they should avoid very bright or reflective colors (e.g., bright whites), as well as reds or oranges (Simpson et al., 2016). Each noted type of clothing has been suggested to interfere with the camera's focus, creating visual issues (Lozano et al., 2015; Simpson et al., 2016). For example, Lozano and colleagues (2015) suggested that highly textured and brightly pattered backgrounds or clothing can create a higher demand for the amount of data that needs to be transmitted, potentially creating slower transmission of information for weaker systems. Nevertheless, on a simpler level, the pattered or bright clothing can be distracting for others, especially for those with attention-related difficulties. In addition to general clothing, the provider and patient should avoid "jangly" or dangling jewelry due to the high likelihood of such accessories being distracting (Lozano et al., 2015; Simpson et al, 2016). Finally, consideration should be given to glasses. For those who wear glasses, monitoring and adjusting may be necessary to avoid light glaring off the lenses into the camera. Further, and more specific to the provider, glasses can accidentally reflect something that the provider does not want the patient to see (e.g., patient notes, a personal belonging off-screen), thus requiring the provider to self-monitor (Simpson et al., 2016).

Before-Session Factors

In efforts to support productive sessions, all users should ensure proper camera setup and lighting (see Chapter 12), turn off unnecessary computer programs, and pre-test their equipment prior to beginning the clinical work (Simpson et al., 2016). This testing should include basic image quality when someone is still, and should also involve people moving their hands and body to ensure the movement is smooth on both ends. This pre-session check is also a good time to ensure that the pan, tilt, and zoom features of a PTZ camera work, if available (Myers et al., 2017). If issues are recognized for any component, this check can allow for parties to problem-solve (e.g., changing video settings, restarting videoconferencing platform, resetting internet) before any important information is discussed. In supplement of basic checks, before beginning, the provider should practice adjusting the videoconferencing platform's settings and video quality features so that they can seamlessly adjust options as needed during session with minimal interruptions. This practice can reduce the provider's need to look away from the screen while making needed adjustments (Lozano et al., 2015; Simpson et al., 2016). Finally, if allowed through the videoconferencing platform, some have suggested the provider and patient should turn off picture-in-picture (PIP) features. While this feature allows the speaker to see themselves in the window, it has been suggested as being distracting (Lozano et al., 2015; Simpson et al., 2016).

During-Session Factors

Once session begins, as further detailed in Chapter 12, the provider should position the video image in a way that will allow one to look at the screen, while capturing their eye gaze in the video camera to simulate direct eye contact (Grayson & Monk, 2003; Simpson et al., 2016; Shore et al., 2018). Following this adjustment to ensure telepresence, the provider should conduct their session as they normally would (i.e., similar content and discussion style), with some additional considerations. While some have suggested using hands and nonverbal behaviors (e.g., head nods) in a similar way as would be done in F2F interactions, others have recommended that providers should slightly exaggerate these motions to ensure they are easily viewed on the videoconferencing image (Lozano et al., 2015). Of note, "slightly exaggerate" means just that, as providers should remain authentic and avoid excessive or overly dramatic mannerisms that could come across as fake or condescending. Further, providers should take care to avoid overly repetitive mannerisms, such as excessive head nodding (Lozano et al., 2015). As session progresses, the provider should ensure that they are not engaging in distracting behaviors that may be outside of their awareness. Such behaviors may include tapping of pens, clicking of pens, spinning of pens, twisting or playing with one's hair, rocking or spinning in a chair, repetitive shaking of legs, cracking of knuckles, and reading of documents outside of the computer screen (Simpson et al., 2016). Each can be distracting, while also potentially fostering feelings of disengagement of the provider for the patient.

Post-Session Factors

At the end of the session, the provider should turn off their video camera. This can help ensure the provider's privacy, and that unintended people do not view materials that the provider may have in view of the camera after the session (e.g., notes or paperwork containing PHI). Unfortunately, a provider who may have back-to-back sessions may think a patient is disconnected, or that another patient has not already connected, but accidentally shows their camera. While such an issue can be partially mitigated through enabling a virtual waiting room, good practice is merely to deactivate the video camera until needed.

Summary Points

- Avoid brightly patterned, striped, checkered, or reflective clothing that could interfere with video quality.
- Avoid bright whites, red, and orange clothing.
- Avoid dangling jewelry.
- Before the session begins, explicitly test the video quality for both the provider and patient, turn off other programs that may consume computer power, and turn off PIP (if possible).
- Providers should become comfortable adjusting the video quality settings, as well as panning, tilting, or zooming (if available), without disruption to session or having to "look away from the patient" for long periods of time.
- During the session, the provider's image should be adjacent to the patient's line of vision to simulate eye contact.
- During the session, the provider should use typical, but slightly exaggerated, hand and facial gestures.
- During the session, all members should avoid fidgeting, rocking, or other distracting movements.
- After the session, the provider should turn their camera off to ensure both provider privacy, and that they do not inadvertently show confidential information.

References

Grayson, D. M., & Monk, A. F. (2003). Are you looking at me? Eye contact and desktop video conferencing. *ACM Transactions on Computer-Human Interaction (TOCHI)*, *10*(3), 221–243. https://doi.org/10.1145/937549.937552.

Lozano, B. E., Birks, A. H., Kloezeman, K., Cha, N., Morland, L. A., & Tuerk, P. W. (2015). Therapeutic alliance in clinical videoconferencing: Optimizing the communication context. In P. W. Tuerk & P. Shore (Eds.), *Clinical videoconferencing in telehealth: Program development and practice* (pp. 221–251). Cham: Springer International.

Luxton, D. D., Pruitt, L. D., & Osenbach, J. E. (2014). Best practices for remote psychological assessment via telehealth technologies. *Professional Psychology: Research and Practice, 45*(1), 27–35. https://doi.org/10.1037/a0034547.

Myers, K., Nelson, E. -L., Rabinowitz, T., Hilty, D., Baker, D., Barnwell, S. S., ... Bernard, J. (2017). American Telemedicine Association practice guidelines for telemental health with children and adolescents. *Telemedicine and e-Health, 23*(10), 779–804. https://doi.org/10.1089/tmj.2017.0177.

Simpson, S., Richardson, L., & Reid, C. (2016). Therapeutic alliance in videoconferencing psychotherapy. In S. Gross, K. Anthony, L. S. Stretch, & D. M. Nagel (Eds.), *Technology in mental health: Applications in practice, supervision, and training* (2nd ed., pp. 99–116). Springfield, IL: Charles C. Thomas.

Shore, J. H., Yellowlees, P., Caudill, R., Johnston, B., Turvey, C., Mishkind, M., ... Hilty, D. (2018). Best practices in videoconferencing telemental health, April 2018. *Telemedicine and e-Health, 24*(11), 827–832. https://doi.org/10.1089/tmj.2018.0237.

14 Videoconferencing Logistics
Audio Tips

As a provider prepares to begin a videoconferencing assessment or treatment session, steps should be taken to ensure the clarity and quality of the audio (Luxton et al., 2016, chap. 2; Myers et al., 2017). Clear audio is needed to not only ensure the building of rapport, but also for the collection of information based on verbal report and auditory observations. The following are audio-related tips to foster an effective and productive session. Tips can be broadly classified as being related to clothing, before-session factors, during-session factors, and post-session factors.

Clothing

While many would consider one's clothing more related to video image, dress can also influence audio. More specifically, the provider should model and encourage the patient to avoid wearing clothing that could create significant noise that interferes with the audio quality. It is important to remember that small noises can be amplified by the microphone, which may be problematic for the distance videoconferencing user. Problematic clothing may include hanging and clanging jewelry (e.g., necklaces, bracelets, or earrings), and materials or fabrics (e.g., leather, velvet, nylon) that create noise (e.g., cracking, rustling, squeaking) when one moves (Simpson et al., 2016).

Before-Session Factors

Prior to the session beginning, the provider should explicitly sound test their microphone, and request a verification and sound test for the patient's location (Simpson et al., 2016). Unfortunately, sometimes someone can be generally heard for single words, but once they start speaking in full sentences or for extended periods, the audio begins to cut in and out. Testing at the onset can help remedy such recognized challenges. To assist in reducing interruptions throughout the session, the provider and patient should turn off other computer programs, as allowed. For example, unless they need to be open for specific reasons, closing email, chat, or reminder programs that will create chimes can reduce noise-based distractions.

Similarly, all phones and devices should be silenced or set to vibrate, if possible (Simpson et al., 2016).

During-Session Factors

Luxton et al. (2014) highlighted that during a session, the audio volume should be loud enough at each end so that everyone can be easily heard, but not so loud that the session can be overheard by others outside of the room. Speaking voice should remain relatively normal in terms of volume and rate; however, one should be mindful of the need to provide frequent pauses to allow for those on the other end of the videoconferencing call to respond. As interrupting can create issues for both the therapeutic alliance and therapeutic outcomes, similar to working with medical interpreters for language differences, the provider should encourage that all members of the session speak in short sentences, and wait a few seconds before speaking again to ensure that the initial speaker is done (e.g., to account for audio lag and if someone is thinking of their next comment; Hadziabdic & Hjelm, 2013; Juckett & Unger, 2014). This notion of waiting before immediately speaking to avoid speaking over each other can be especially important for videoconferencing, as some microphones and software will cut the sound of a second speaker if someone is already speaking, thus resulting in missed information (Simpson et al., 2016). Finally, to avoid disruptions during session, the provider and patient should be careful to avoid any noises that may be amplified by a microphone. Such activities could include typing on a keyboard, rustling papers, or writing on hard surfaces (Simpson et al., 2016).

Post-Session Factors

It is important for the provider to mute their microphone at the end of the session. This can ensure that inadvertent discussion or comments are not captured by the microphone for any unintended audience (Simpson et al., 2016). This is especially important for providers who read documents out loud to themselves, make phone calls, or speak to colleagues between sessions.

Summary Points

- Ensure that the provider and patient avoid clothing that will create distracting noise throughout a session.
- Before the session begins, the provider and patient should explicitly test the audio quality, turn off other programs that may create noise, and silence any phones or other devices.
- During the session, the provider and patient should speak at a normal volume and rate, but consider speaking in shorter sentences, and

providing a few extra seconds after sentences to help reduce speaking over each other.

- During the session, the provider and patient should avoid engaging in activities that may be amplified through a microphone. These activities include typing, rustling papers, or writing on hard surfaces.
- When the session is completed, the provider should mute their microphone to ensure no transmission of unintended information.

References

Hadziabdic, E., & Hjelm, K. (2013). Working with interpreters: Practical advice for use of an interpreter in healthcare. *International Journal of Evidence-Based Healthcare, 11*(1), 69–76. https://doi.org/10.1111/1744-1609.12005.

Juckett, G., & Unger, K. (2014). Appropriate use of medical interpreters. *American Family Physician, 90*(7), 476–480.

Luxton, D. D., Nelson, E. -L., & Maheu, M. M. (2016). *A practitioner's guide to telemental health: How to conduct legal, ethical, and evidence-based telepractice.* Washington, DC: American Psychological Association.

Luxton, D. D., Pruitt, L. D., & Osenbach, J. E. (2014). Best practices for remote psychological assessment via telehealth technologies. *Professional Psychology: Research and Practice, 45*(1), 27–35. https://doi.org/10.1037/a0034547.

Myers, K., Nelson, E. -L., Rabinowitz, T., Hilty, D., Baker, D., Barnwell, S. S., … Bernard, J. (2017). American Telemedicine Association practice guidelines for telemental health with children and adolescents. *Telemedicine and e-Health, 23*(10), 779–804. https://doi.org/10.1089/tmj.2017.0177.

Simpson, S., Richardson, L., & Reid, C. (2016). Therapeutic alliance in videoconferencing psychotherapy. In S. Gross, K. Anthony, L. S. Stretch, & D. M. Nagel (Eds.), *Technology in mental health: Applications in practice, supervision, and training* (2nd ed., pp. 99–116). Springfield, IL: Charles C. Thomas.

15 Videoconferencing Logistics

Documentation

Whether via paper charts or an EHR, the provider's sessions must be documented and placed into the patient's record. This practice is as true for videoconferencing as it is for F2F encounters. As the use of the technology adds additional and unique considerations, the provider should take care to document these aspects to accurately reflect all parts of the session's content (Maheu et al., 2001, chap. 9; Smucker Barnwell et al., 2018). While dozens of articles, book chapters, and guidebooks detail the necessity of documenting the videoconferencing-specific aspects, focused guidance on what to include and how to include it has been relatively minimal. Due to this, the following are suggestions to assist providers in documenting videoconferencing-based work. Suggestions are meant as template materials, as each practice will be unique, thus requiring tailoring. To supplement the following information, providers should contact their licensing boards and insurance panels in order to inquire about details that are recommended for inclusion in the documentation. Ultimately, one's unique practice and documentation preferences should guide the creation of a formal documentation scheme.

General Factors to Include

When documenting a videoconferencing encounter, the provider should initially include all pertinent information that they would provide for a typical F2F note. Such information may include the patient's name and identifying information (e.g., medical record number), dates and times of session, direct patient contact time, participants, diagnoses, treatment goals and plans, mental status, risk assessment, and the session content itself, including objective and subjective data (e.g., therapy session information, assessment information, diagnostic conceptualization; Luxton et al., 2016, chap. 6; Maheu et al., 2001, chap. 9). Supplemental information would then relate to the videoconferencing processes. In no particular order, these details include: the rationale for the videoconferencing being used, platforms used, if issues were recognized with the platform and how they were remedied, provider location details (i.e., distant site information), patient location details (i.e., originating site information), a statement of ongoing appropriateness of the videoconferencing for the patient, a statement of verification of the patient's identity, and potential emergency contact information. Where the provider places such information in the note is up to them. It can be included as a built-in narrative to the session's general content, or can be in a "telehealth" or "videoconferencing-specific" section. See Figure 15.1 for an example of compiled information.

Rationale for Videoconferencing Being Rendered

A provider should detail the reasons why videoconferencing was used in replacement of the more traditional F2F interactions. This is true whether the patient seems like an appropriate candidate, or if videoconferencing was selected due to other options being limited for a high-risk patient (Shore & Lu, 2015; Smucker Barwell et al., 2018). For example, if videoconferencing was chosen due to the patient living several hours away without local options, a statement could read:

> Videoconferencing was utilized due to [patient name] living approximately [distance] from the provider, and no similar services being available in [his/her] vicinity. Videoconferencing allowed the provider and [patient name] an ability to both see and hear each other in real time.

Alternatively, if the patient is within a near vicinity of providers, but has physical mobility issues precluding them from attending F2F care, a statement could read:

> Videoconferencing services were rendered due to [patient name] being physically unable to attend face-to-face services as a result of a physical disability reducing mobility. Videoconferencing services allowed the provider and [patient name] an ability to both see and hear each other in real time.

Finally, should the videoconferencing be indicated due to a natural disaster or event, such as the 2020 COVID-19 pandemic, a statement could read:

> Videoconferencing was utilized due to the provider and [patient name]'s desire to adhere to CDC [Centers for Disease Control and Prevention] and US government recommendations suggesting the limiting of face-to-face services in efforts to reduce the spread of COVID-19. Videoconferencing allowed the provider and [patient name] an ability to both see and hear each other in real time.

Platforms Used

The provider may also wish to list which videoconferencing platform was utilized, including an indication of whether the platform identifies itself as

Telehealth procedures

Rationale for telehealth-based services:
Videoconferencing was utilized due to Jim Doe living approximately four
  hours from the provider and no similar services being available in his vicinity.
  Videoconferencing allowed the provider and Jim an ability to both see and hear
  each other in real time.

Telecommunication platform(s) used:
Super Videoconferencing

**(If videoconferencing) Is telecommunication platform HIPAA compliant (e.g., at
  least 128-bit encryption, BAA signed)?**
Yes

(If videoconferencing) Any issues/interruptions with technology throughout session?
Yes. Poor connection resulted in limited high-definition video, and created audio
  issues for both the provider and Jim. The provider attempted to address issues
  for approximately two minutes, in which time the provider and Jim reconnected
  to the videoconferencing platform. Reconnection remedied issues and session
  progressed without additional interruption.

Provider distant site location:
Address: 123 Psychology Avenue, Fort Lauderdale, FL 33322
Location: Psychological Practice and Associates; Office 4

Patient/family reported originating site location:
Name: Jim Doe
Phone number: 123-123-1234
Email: 123@email.com
Address: 1234 Blue Street, Gainesville, FL 32601
Location: home; private room with only Jim and his wife being present

Identity verification:
Identity of Jim Doe was verified via state-issued photo identification held to the
  video camera

Alternative contact information:
Name: Jane Doe
Relationship: patient's wife
Phone Number: 123-123-1235
Email: 125@email.com
Address: 1234 Blue Street, Gainesville, FL 32601

Local/nearest medical center information provided by patient/family:
Name: Blue Hospital
Phone number: 123-987-9876
Address: 456 Blue Street, Gainesville, FL 32601

Local/nearest law enforcement information provided by patient/family:
Name: Blue Police Department
Phone number: 123-456-4567
Address: 258 Red Street, Gainesville, FL 32601

Figure 15.1 Sample videoconferencing-specific information that could be included
  in the session note (block format)*.
Note: * Information provided is meant for demonstration purposes only and should be modified for the provider's practice.

HIPAA compliant. This could be as simple as indicating, "[Platform name] was used for the videoconferencing session," or can be more detailed, such as,

> [Platform name] was used for the videoconferencing session. The platform was indicated to provide [level of encryption], and a business associates agreement (BAA) was secured that was signed by both [the provider or provider's company] and the videoconferencing platform company.

If Issues Were Recognized with the Platform and How They Were Remedied

Given the potential for technology-based interruptions to sessions, the provider should detail whether issues were recognized throughout the care. This is potentially as simple as indicating, "No issues with the videoconferencing platform were recognized throughout the session." If issues were to arise, the provider should supply enough detail to indicate how impactful the interruption was on the session content. For example, the provider could detail issues in a manner similar to the following:

> Poor connection resulted in limited high-definition video, and created audio issues for both the provider and [patient name]. The provider attempted to address issues for approximately [time in minutes], in which time the provider and [patient name] reconnected to the videoconferencing platform, and adjusted settings to facilitate improved video and audio quality. This was effective, with session continuing uninterrupted.

Should issues continue even after attempts to reconnect and change the settings, instead of indicating that the approach was effective, a provider could instead document,

> "As a result of these strategies failing, the backup HIPAA-compliant, agreed-upon videoconferencing platform, [platform name], was utilized. This second platform functioned appropriately without issue. The session was interrupted for approximately four minutes."

Finally, if all videoconferencing platforms fail (e.g., full internet connection failure), and a provider must switch modalities to a back-up agreed-upon means, they could detail the entire scenario, such as:

> Poor connection resulted in limited high-definition video, and created audio issues for both the provider and [patient name]. The provider attempted to address issues for approximately [time in minutes], in which time the provider and [patient name] reconnected to the videoconferencing platform, and adjusted settings to facilitate improved

video and audio quality. As a result of this failing, the backup HIPAA-compliant, agreed-upon videoconferencing platform, [platform name], was utilized. This second platform also proved insufficient, prompting the provider to [back-up plan, such as using a telephone call]. This back-up proved successful and session continued without additional interruption. The total amount of time lost was [time in minutes].

Provider Location Details (i.e., Distant Site Information)

As is often suggested by those who study and practice telehealth, such as videoconferencing (e.g., Luxton et al., 2016, chap. 6; Maheu et al., 2001, chap. 9), the provider should detail their location of practice as an indication of the distant site. To supply such information, the provider can indicate the location of their practice in name (e.g., the company, practice, clinic, university, or medical center), as well as the specific office or room if in a larger center (e.g., "Office 4 of Psychological Practice and Associates"). The provider may also consider providing the full address of where the practice occurred to detail the physical location of the distant site provider.

Patient Location Details (i.e., Originating Site Information)

In addition to the distant site information, the provider should detail the patient's location. This documents the originating site and can help verify that the patient was in a location of the provider's license (Luxton et al., 2016, chap. 6; Maheu et al., 2001, chap. 9). Such information can include general contact information (e.g., phone number, email), the type of setting (e.g., home, car, private room in patient's location of employment), the full address, and an indication of who was present in the room. For example, as based upon information provided by the patient, the provider may document that,

> "[Patient name] reported that they were in their [name of state] home in a private room with only [patient name] and [his/her] [other members] being present and participating."

If children are in the room, but not involved in the session, the provider may indicate,

> "Due to the need to care for young children, the session also included [insert additional individuals]. The children played on the floor and did not actively participate in session."

If the patient had to use a location that may not be ideal, but was the only possible option at the time, the provider should indicate such through the documentation:

While [patient name] reportedly attempted to utilize [his/her] bedroom as had been used for prior sessions, family visiting the home precluded this. [Patient name] indicated that the only private place in the home was [his/her] bathroom. While comfort-based and potential camera view-based limitations were discussed, this location was agreed upon by the provider and patient.

Statement of Ongoing Appropriateness of Videoconferencing for Patient

In efforts to ensure ongoing safe and ethical care, the provider can indicate in the documentation that they have an ongoing evaluation of the patient (Luxton et al., 2016, chap. 6; Smucker Barnwell et al., 2018). This evaluation should consider not only the patient's emotional and behavioral status, but general risks, adherence to medication regimen if pertinent, physical ability, and other stressors that may impede therapeutic processes. In doing so, the provider can document that they had been proactive in ensuring safe and effective videoconferencing care. This statement can be built into the clinical session summary narrative by indicating:

> "As based upon [observations of clinical presentation in sessions, self-reported status, rating scales], [patient name] appeared to have minimal risk and continues to present as an acceptable candidate for videoconferencing services."

Should the patient present with a concern that may lead to the provider pausing or terminating videoconferencing, documentation could read:

> Due to [patient name]'s reported [increase in challenging behaviors or risk-related factors, difficulty finding a private space for the videoconferencing sessions, technological issues that preclude the videoconferencing sessions], the provider and patient discussed the provider's concerns with ongoing videoconferencing. It was collaboratively decided that due to recognized issues, the use of distance videoconferencing will be paused in favor of [alternatives such as F2F visits, telephone calls]. Use of videoconferencing will be re-evaluated as based upon need and appropriateness as sessions progress.

Statement of Verification of the Patient's Identity

As providers should verify the patient's identity prior to discussing any confidential information, especially if an initial session without a prior F2F meeting, such processes should be documented (Luxton et al., 2016, chap. 6). Such documentation could be brief and read:

> "Identity of [patient name] was verified via state-issued photo identification held to the video camera."

Emergency Contact Information

Providers should always have emergency contacts and an emergency plan available when conducting videoconferencing, as one never knows what may occur (APA, 2013; Gamble et al., 2015; Shore & Lu, 2015; Smucker Barnwell et al., 2018). If the information is readily available in their full medical record, a statement could read:

> Emergency contact information including the address, phone number, and email for [patient name], alternative contacts, the nearest medical center, and the nearest law enforcement center were gathered at the onset of treatment and are available in [patient name]'s medical record.

While not essential, the provider may alternatively include such emergency contact directly into the individual note if it is easier to locate should the medical charting or EHR be more complex and take time to sift through to find the necessary information.

Initial Contact-Specific Documentation

While all aforementioned detail should be considered for inclusion in any general videoconferencing documentation note, when conducting an initial contact and collecting informed consent, additional information should be recorded. This information should clearly indicate that the provider considered multiple factors and took necessary ethical and legal steps prior to beginning full videoconferencing services. Information can be separated by content. First is an indication of why videoconferencing was selected for the specific patient. This statement can be near identical to those listed in the "Rationale for Videoconferencing Being Rendered" section, or modified with more detail for the individual's unique situation. For example,

> Videoconferencing will be utilized for future sessions due to [patient name] living approximately [distance] from the provider and no similar services being available in [his/her] vicinity. Videoconferencing services will allow the provider and [patient name] an ability to both see and hear each other in real time.

Second should be an indication that the patient was screened for appropriateness. An example of this could read:

> Prior to the provider and [patient name] agreeing on videoconferencing services, [patient name] was screened for appropriateness as based upon several factors that align with the American Psychological Association and American Telemedicine Association recommendations, including [patient name]'s technological knowledge and attitudes, past experiences with both mental health and technology-enhanced

treatments, availability of appropriate videoconferencing technology, diagnostic considerations, physical disabilities or limitations, access to F2F providers, and possibility for safety concerns.

While this information can be modified and shortened, it is meant to convey that the provider is not only aware of the literature guiding appropriateness, but that they did their due diligence to screen the patients for the videoconferencing. Third, the provider should clearly document the informed consent and safety planning processes (described in Chapter 4). This detailing may include a general statement that informed consent information was reviewed and the patient provided their consent, or can include specific detail of what was covered as part of the informed consent process. An example of the more specific detailing could read,

> [Patient name] signed a telehealth-specific informed consent form that detailed pertinent information, including strengths and limitations of the approach, scheduling information, payment details, and communication strategies between sessions, as well as an emergency contact form that included the local hospital and law enforcement office of [patient name] to plan for any potential crises. [Patient name] also agreed to update the provider prior to the onset of the session should [he/she] ever be out of the state of the provider's license. See medical record for copies of paperwork. Information was also provided verbally.

Fourth, while not essential, it may be prudent to include a statement that the provider will supply the videoconferencing as long as it is helpful and safe. Should the services no longer be reasonable, optimal, or safe, the provider has the right to cease the videoconferencing services in favor of a more beneficial and/or safe alternative. This clause could read:

> It was discussed that if at any time the provider believes that the videoconferencing method is no longer effective or beneficial, or if there is an increased potential for harm to [patient name] or another individual as a result of the continued videoconferencing, alternatives will be discussed, with referrals provided as necessary.

Finally, the provider may wish to document that a safety word/phrase (detailed in Chapter 4) was created. See Figure 15.2 for an integrated summary of such information.

Assessment-Specific Modifications

If a provider is to be conducting psychoeducational, psychological, or neuropsychological assessments, while much of the aforementioned documentation components remain relevant, additional specification and modification should be made to clarify the process of the assessments through videoconferencing. As an example, the provider can begin the assessment

(a) To align with CDC/WHO/US government regulation suggesting social distancing to reduce the chances of COVID-19 spread, the provider and patient collaboratively agreed to conduct sessions via videoconferencing. (b) Prior to the provider and Mr. Smith's agreement of videoconferencing, Mr. Smith was screened for appropriateness as based upon several factors that align with the American Psychological Association and American Telemedicine Association recommendations, including Mr. Smith's technological knowledge and attitudes, past experiences with both mental health and technology-enhanced treatments, availability of appropriate videoconferencing technology, diagnostic considerations, physical disabilities or limitations, access to F2F providers, and possibility for safety concerns. (c) Mr. Smith signed a telehealth-specific informed consent sheet that detailed pertinent information including strengths and limitations of the approach, scheduling information, payment details, and communication strategies between sessions, as well as an emergency contact sheet that included the local hospital and law enforcement office of Mr. Smith to plan for any potential crises. Mr. Smith also agreed to update the provider prior to the onset of the session should he ever be out of the state of the provider's license. See medical record for copies of paperwork. This information was also provided verbally. (d) In addition to logistics that were detailed in the signed forms, it was discussed that if at any time the provider believes that the videoconferencing method is no longer effective or beneficial, or if there is an increased potential for harm to Mr. Smith or another as a result of continued videoconferencing, alternatives will be discussed, with referrals provided as necessary. (e) A safety word/phrase of "banana" was created and agreed to, should services need to be ended due to an issue arising, or an unauthorized participating listening into or joining the session.**

Figure 15.2 Sample videoconferencing statement for introductory note*.

Notes: * Information provided is meant for demonstration purposes only and should be modified for the provider's practice.

** (a) Rationale for videoconferencing services being rendered; (b) patient screening processes; (c) informed consenting and safety planning processes; (d) disclaimer of the provider's right to cease videoconferencing services if they are deemed inappropriate or harmful; (e) creation of safety word/phrase.

documentation with a clear description of why the assessment was conducted through videoconferencing instead of the more traditional F2F method. This statement can be identical to or slightly modified from those listed in the "Rationale for Videoconferencing Being Rendered" section:

> "Due to [patient name] being unable to secure psychological assessment within [distance] of [his/her] home, it was collaboratively agreed that the assessment will be completed through videoconferencing." This can be followed by an indication of where the assessment processes occurred, such as in the patient's home, or a local clinic. For instance, "[Patient name] was interviewed in the living room of their home in Chicago, Illinois" or "[Patient name] was interviewed in a private room at their local primary care provider's office in Chicago. Illinois."

To document that the provider ensured that the interviewee was the appropriate patient, the identify verification should be detailed, with verbiage that can match those discussed in the "Statement of Verification of the Patient's Identity" section. Following this information, the provider can include statements indicating that the patient agreed to not record the assessment processes, that they completed the assessment in a private and secure room, and that no one interrupted or coached them. This can be completed by having a direct statement on each, such as:

> [Patient name] agreed that no one would record any of the assessment sessions. [He/she] indicated that the room of the assessment was secure and private. Based on report and observation, no one interrupted the assessment session, and [patient's name] did not have to use a safety word/phrase to indicate that [he/she] was being observed or coerced into providing false information. Review of video footage validated reports of independent completion.

A clear indication of how the assessment was completed should then be included, with a statement regarding whether it was through screen sharing, multiple camera setup, or another means. A sample of this may read:

> "The [type of assessment] included [name of measures], and were proctored through the use of [methodology such as the use of screen-sharing technology, multiple camera setups]."

If relevant, the provider can also indicate that use of the videoconferencing does not violate the measure's terms of use. Finally, as based upon the provider's knowledge as to whether the specific assessments have been empirically supported for use through videoconferencing, as well as expected differences of outcomes (e.g., if normative data aren't available for distance administration, latency issues limiting clinical utility), an indication should be given as to the provider's judgment of whether the assessment is an accurate representation of the patient's true abilities. All of this information can be documented through statements that read:

> The [psychoeducational/psychological/neuropsychological] assessment materials utilized have been empirically evaluated with outcomes suggesting that the findings were equivalent when administered online to what would be obtained from a F2F pencil-and-paper administration. As based upon this information and observations, it is the provider's professional clinical judgment that the data obtained from the assessment is appropriate and generally equivalent to what would have been obtained if [patient name] had completed the assessment in-person.

See Figure 15.3 for an integrated summary of such information.

(a) Due to Mrs. White being unable to secure psychological assessment within four hours of her home, it was collaboratively agreed that the assessment will be completed through videoconferencing. (b) Mrs. White was interviewed in her home-based office in Naperville, Illinois. (c) Her identity was verified through her holding a government-issues passport to the video camera. (d) Mrs. White agreed that no one will record any of the assessment sessions. She indicated that the room was secure and private. Based on report and observation, no one interrupted the assessment, and Mrs. White did not have to use a safety word/phrase to indicate that she was being observed or coerced into providing false information. Review of video footage validated reports of independent completion. (e) The psychological assessments included [insert measure names], and were proctored through the provider's use of screen sharing of the material to Mrs. White through the videoconferencing platform. This approach was deemed acceptable per the assessment measure's terms of use and copyright agreements. (f) The psychological assessment materials utilized have been empirically evaluated with outcomes suggesting that the findings were equivalent when administered online to what would be obtained from a F2F pencil-and-paper administration. As based upon this information and observations, it is the provider's professional clinical judgment that the data obtained from the assessment is appropriate and generally equivalent to what would have been obtained if Mrs. Smith had completed the assessment in person.**

Figure 15.3 Sample videoconferencing statement for assessment note*.

Source: The clause is an adaptation of one created by R. Kaplan (personal communication, April 17, 2020).

Notes: * Information provided is meant for demonstration purposes only and should be modified for the provider's practice.

** (a) Rationale for videoconferencing assessment process; (b) location of assessment; (c) identity verification process; (d) privacy indication; (e) assessment administration process; (f) statement of assessment validity.

Summary Points

- When conducting videoconferencing, the provider should supplement their typical session documentation with videoconferencing-specific details.
- Related to the videoconferencing-focused components, providers should considering detailing the rationale for the videoconferencing being used instead of traditional F2F methods, platforms used, if issues were recognized with the platform and how they were remedied, details of the provider's location (i.e., distant site information), details of the patient's location (i.e., originating site information), a statement of ongoing appropriateness of the videoconferencing for the patient, a statement of verification of the patient's identity, and emergency contact information.
- For initial contact documentation, the provider should consider detailing not only the rationale for the videoconferencing being rendered in replace of F2F care, but also the appropriateness screening processes of the patient, the informed consent and safety planning

processes, the creation of a safety word or phrase, and possibly an indication that videoconferencing methods can be terminated at any time with alternatives being presented should the provider deem them unsuitable for the patient.

- For assessment sessions, the provider should consider detailing the rationale for the videoconferencing assessment processes being rendered instead of F2F services, the location of the assessment, the identify verification processes, notice of the patient completing the assessment independently in a private location, the actual assessment administration processes and how they were delivered, and statements regarding the assessment's perceived validity and reliability as based upon the measure itself (e.g., research supporting distance use, normative data for digital administration) and the patient's performance.

References

American Psychological Association (APA). (2013). *Guidelines for the practice of telepsychology.* Retrieved from www.apa.org/practice/guidelines/telepsychology.

Gamble, N., Boyle, C., & Morris, Z. A. (2015). Ethical practice in telepsychology. *Australian Psychologist, 50*(4), 292–298. https://doi.org/10.1111/ap.12133.

Luxton, D. D., Nelson, E. -L., & Maheu, M. M. (2016). *A practitioner's guide to telemental health: How to conduct legal, ethical, and evidence-based telepractice.* Washington, DC: American Psychological Association.

Maheu, M. M., Whitten, P., & Allen, A. (2001). *e-Health, telehealth, and telemedicine: A guide to start-up and success.* San Francisco, CA: Jossey-Bass.

Shore, P., & Lu, M. (2015). Patient safety planning and emergency management. In P. W. Tuerk & P. Shore (Eds.), *Clinical videoconferencing in telehealth: Program development and practice* (pp. 167–201). Cham: Springer International.

Smucker Barnwell, S., McCann, R., & McCutcheon, S. (2018). Competence of the psychologist. In L. F. Campbell, F. Millán, & J. N. Martin (Eds.), *A telepsychology casebook: Using technology ethically and effectively in your professional practice* (pp. 7–26). Washington, DC: American Psychological Association.

16 A Stepwise Summary of the Videoconferencing Process

As the use of videoconferencing can be quite complex with numerous individual components, the following is a stepwise summary and consolidation of information presented in prior chapters related to both the setup and implementation. In supplement of this summary, providers may find additional assistance through a more detailed overview of processes presented in Appendix H, as well as practice-oriented videoconferencing checklists presented in Appendices I and J.

Setting Up the Videoconferencing Processes

Through the consolidation of information, five key processes can be viewed as important when setting up a videoconferencing service for patient care. This remains true whether the service is assessment-based or intervention-focused.

1. *Verification of the appropriateness of the patient and setting.* Patient factors must be assessed to ensure that services can be provided in an effective and safe manner. Related to the patient themselves, consideration should be given to numerous factors, including, but not limited to, history with and attitudes towards mental health services and technology, diagnoses, behavioral risk, available technology, barriers to F2F or technology-based care (e.g., financial, transportation, physical disability), support systems should a crisis occur, and general levels of motivation for the mental health services. Related to setting, the location should be private, quiet, and uncluttered; have minimal distractions; and foster minimal interruptions. Ideal settings have the provider's and patient's location appear similar to a normal office setting in order to recreate a professional atmosphere.
2. *Gathering of verbal and written informed consent.* To ensure that the patient understands the videoconferencing processes and is able to provide informed consent, they should have time to review the full informed consent forms, and participate in a discussion in which the provider reviews the information and answers any questions. The process should cover indications of general practice including what

types of services will be offered; strengths and limitations of video-conferencing; delivery factors including how videoconferencing differ from F2F care; communication considerations including appropriate means of contact and turn-around times for phone calls or emails; and administrative policies such as billing, scheduling, and documentation. The process not only helps a patient to decide about participation, but helps set reasonable expectations for both what will occur, and the outcomes to expect.

3. *Gathering of emergency contacts.* Regardless of whether a patient presents as high or minimal risk, providers considering videoconferencing should have a concrete safety plan for each patient. As part of this process, before services begin, the provider should gather information including the patient's full contact information (i.e., address, email, phone number), alternative names and contact information (e.g., family members, spouses, community members that can assist in emergency situations), name and contact information for the nearest medical center, name and contact information for the nearest law enforcement office, criteria for what is considered an emergency situation, steps to take in order to ensure a safe environment, a plan should the patient be unable to get into contact with the provider, and an indication that the plan was reviewed and agreed to by both the patient and the provider. Such information should be maintained in a readily accessible location, should an emergency arise.

4. *Detailing of a plan for technology-related issues.* Building upon what is discussed throughout the informed consent process, additional detail should be provided for session-to-session management of technology-related issues. The provider should detail what steps to take and alternatives that may be used when technological issues arise. In addition to basic problem-solving (e.g., restarting the services), the plan may include the use of a secondary, back-up video-conferencing platform, as well as the use of other methods (e.g., telephone).

5. *Creating a safety word or phrase.* As issues may arise that require an immediate termination of the videoconferencing session, the provider and patient should establish a safety word or phrase that would cue the provider to immediately end the videoconferencing call. While reasons for use may vary by patient (e.g., other members of the household not knowing that the individual is receiving psychological services), availability of a safety word or phrase can increase the patient's perceived safety and comfort throughout the therapeutic processes.

Conducting the Videoconferencing Sessions

Through the consolidation of information, ten key processes can be viewed as important when conducting videoconferencing.

1. *Testing the equipment prior to beginning session.* Before the session even begins, the equipment should be tested for both the provider's and patient's end to ensure that everything is working properly. As part of this process, providers may use the preview or test-calling features of many videoconferencing platforms to explicitly test the video and audio. Additionally, the provider can use online tools to more directly access bandwidth and latency to ensure that both are appropriate for the videoconferencing services.

2. *Sending links to the videoconferencing platform.* Whether using a static (i.e., unchanging) weblink to join the videoconferencing platform, or if needing to send a unique link and password for every session, such information should be sent to the patient in advance of the session so that they can easily find it and connect with ample time. This is especially important for initial meetings where the patient may have to download drivers, updates, or programs to allow for the videoconferencing platform to work. Links should be sent through encrypted emails to ensure privacy of information.

3. *Providing documentation.* If a provider is aware of the content of the session (e.g., a specific CBT skill, a specific topic of parent management training) and has handouts to supplement discussions, the provider can create a means to share such documentation. One method is to send the handouts prior to session through an encrypted email or file-sharing program so that the document can be reviewed by the patient before, during, and/or following the session. Alternatively, some videoconferencing platforms allow for files to be securely shared and downloaded through the platform itself. If files cannot be shared, or the provider was not aware of what was going to be covered in session, screen sharing can allow the provider to project the documents of their display screen to the patient's view.

4. *Verifying video and audio quality.* Once the videoconferencing session begins, the provider should verify the patient's video and audio connection before asking the patient to verify the provider's quality on their end.

5. *Closing other programs and silencing all devices.* At the onset of the videoconferencing session, in addition to asking that the patient silence any phones or other devices, the provider should ask the patient to close any other unnecessary programs or apps on their system. This is done not only to save power for weaker systems, but can also help avoid interruptions that may come from program-related pop-ups (e.g., reminders).

6. *Verifying identities.* Before discussing any confidential information, especially for the initial sessions, the patient's identity should be verified. This can help ensure that only appropriate individuals are part of the videoconferencing sessions and are privy to confidential information. Holding a photo identification (e.g., license, passport) to the video camera can be a simple and helpful method of verifying identities.

7. *Confirming location.* In addition to the verification of identities, the location of the patient should be confirmed. This is important to ensure that the provider is practicing in the states they are licensed in, and to ensure that the patient is in a private space conducive to the videoconferencing work.

8. *Confirming privacy.* Supplementing the physical location itself is the need to confirm the privacy of the session content. First, the provider should verify that either the patient is alone in the room, or that only authorized individuals are present with them. Second, the room should be verified as a location that minimizes the ability for others outside of the room to see or hear the session.

9. *Conducting the session.* Once the session is set up and all aspects are reviewed, the provider will conduct the session. While content may be similar to F2F practices, the provider should consider the differences for the videoconferencing work, including the potential need for slightly exaggerated nonverbal behaviors.

10. *Documenting the session.* Following the session, the provider should document the contact. In addition to any typical documentation that is produced from a F2F encounter, the provider should document videoconferencing-specific information.

17 Self-Care Practices

While not an often-discussed topic within the videoconferencing or broader telehealth literature, the frequent and prolonged use of video-conferencing can create a range of potential physical and ocular health issues for providers. Physical issues can include shoulder, back, neck, elbow, knee, and leg pains associated with inappropriate design or use of furniture, posture issues, and problematic placement of one's wrists, legs, or feet (Shikdar & Al-Kindi, 2007). Ocular issues can be classified under the phrase computer vision syndrome (CVS), which can result from prolonged digital screen exposure (e.g., computers, tablets, smartphones) and include eyestrain, headaches, blurred vision, eye redness, burning sensation, ocular pain, and dry eyes (Turgut, 2018). While each symptom may occur, eyestrain has been suggested as the most common complaint among those viewing screens for six or more hours a day (e.g., videoconferencing sessions with in-between checking of smartphone or email), and can be associated with screen placement, angles, lighting/brightness, and glare (Agarwal et al., 2013). A lack of awareness of either physical or ocular factors for the technology usage has been suggested to predispose users to a range of musculoskeletal and visual disorders. This remains true even for healthcare workers, who have been suggested as being aware of many of the physical and ocular considerations, but infrequently implement self-care principles (Sanaeinasab et al., 2018).

Physical and ocular issues contributed to what many have colloquially referred to as "Zoom fatigue." This form of fatigue results from extended use of any videoconferencing platform, even if it is not Zoom (Sklar, 2020). It is believed to be caused by the provider's inability to use the full range of nonverbal signals and cues that are typically used in F2F encounters, an over-reliance on limited signals and cues that come from watching other people's faces through the videoconferencing platform, needing to maintain a fixed position to ensure that the provider remains in frame of the camera, potentially using equipment that is too small and requires squinting (e.g., smartphone screen), reduced eye blinking that comes from the technology usage, nonstop concentration that is believed to come from being unable to get off camera, and a potential self-consciousness and ongoing evaluation of oneself during videoconferencing (Maheu, 2020).

Table 17.1 Helpful workstation setup resources

Organization	Resource	Link
Occupational Safety and Health Administration (OSHA)	Computer Workstations e-Tool	www.osha.gov/SLTC/etools/computerworkstations/index.html
University of Western Australia	Computer Workstation Ergonomics	www.safety.uwa.edu.au/topics/physical/ergonomics/workstation

To address noted issues, as well as to reduce Zoom fatigue, organizations and researchers of computer ergonomics (a science that focuses on posture and comfort when using computer-based technology), have created recommendations. As based on such works, several key considerations for workstation setup can be highlighted related to the prevention and reduction of issues caused by extended use of videoconferencing. Please see Table 17.1 for additional resources for workstation setup.

Physical Strategies for Self-Care

On the simplest level, a provider should make attempts to limit the amount of continuous time spent in front of a screen without physically moving, whether for the actual videoconferencing session, or for post-session typing of notes (Tribley et al., 2011). To accomplish this, the provider should take standing or walking breaks every 45–60 minutes to help stay loose (Occupational Safety and Health Administration [OSHA], n.d.; Tribley et al., 2011). To further facilitate this, providers can engage in nonvideoconferencing activities requiring physical movement. For example, walking to get a drink of water, walking to throw out papers, going to the restroom, and avoiding eating lunch at one's desk can all get the provider up and moving. Between such physical breaks, providers should frequently adjust their body during the sessions through moving of their legs, knees, arms, elbows, trunk, and neck (Cook & Burgess-Limerick, 2003; OSHA, n.d.). Even if adjusted slightly, it can help reduce issues related to remaining in the same position for too long. If the provider is finding it difficult to engage in strategies or leave their office area, they can also consider adjusting their desk to allow for standing, or purchasing a standing desk that can adjust to the desired height of the provider at different times (Cook & Burgess-Limerick, 2003).

Regarding the arrangement of one's body to maximize physical health, whether sitting at a desk for the session itself or for post-session documentation work, the provider should take care of all major body parts to avoid pains and aches (Figure 17.1). As detailed by Cook and Burgess-Limerick (2003), and OSHA (n.d.), a branch of the US Department of Labor, the provider should seek to have the display screen at approximately eye level to avoid having to dramatically tilt one's head up or down, which may increase neck pain over time. The provider should also seek a chair that supplies back support that conforms to the natural "S" curvature of the provider's spine, with appropriate lumbar support that prevents the ability to slouch. Through sitting in this position, one's shoulders should be relaxed with the upper arms hanging normally at the side of the body throughout session, and with elbows bent between a 90- to 120-degree angle when typing notes or other documentation. A provider's feet should be fully supported either by the floor or a footrest without hanging in the air. Finally, the provider should adjust their chair so that their knees are at about the same height as their hips with their feet slightly forward.

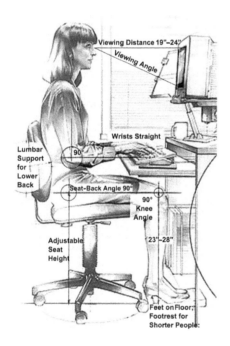

Figure 17.1 Appropriate videoconferencing workstation setup.

Source: Image from Computer Workstation Variables cleanup.png (https://upload. wikimedia.org/wikipedia/commons/c/c0/Computer_Workstation_Variables_ cleanup.png) by Yamavu (August 1, 2013) (https://commons.wikimedia.org/ wiki/User:Yamavu) is licensed under CCO 1.0 (https://creativecommons.org/ publicdomain/zero/1.0/deed.en).

Ocular Strategies for Self-Care

To prevent ocular issues, the provider should enact both physical equipment-related changes and self-changes. First, providers should ensure that the screen is at approximately eye-level (i.e., slightly downward; 4–6 inches below the straight-ahead gaze), and placed at least 20–25 inches (e.g., approximately one's arm length) from one's eyes (Turgut, 2018). Further, one should evaluate the role of glare, reflection, and dust of the screens. For example, glare and dust can impair one's ability to focus, creating eyestrain (Cook & Burgess-Limerick, 2003; Tribley et al., 2011). Frequent cleaning of the screen can help with this. Related to glare and reflection, while simply repositioning the display screen can sometimes address the issues, another option is using a matte screen glare filter to simply block the glare altogether (Turgut, 2018). To further reduce eyestrain and other ocular issues, the provider can increase the contrast of the screen either through manual settings; or by activating a high-contrast mode built into many computer, tablet, or smartphone systems (Turgut, 2018). This can help better differentiate aspects and colors of the images presented on the user's screen.

Related to self-changes, the provider should enact a 20-20-20 rule to briefly rest their eyes either during or between sessions (American Optometric Association [AOA], n.d.; Tribley et al., 2011; Turgut, 2018). In doing so, the provider will take a break every approximately 20 minutes to look away at an object 20 feet away for approximately 20 seconds. Either in replacement of, or in supplement of, the AOA (n.d.) has recommended a break for 15 minutes once every two hours of continuous screen time. To further improve a provider's experience, it is recommended that they make an overt effort to increase the amount of blinking they take. This is in response to findings suggesting that focusing on a screen reduces the amount of blinking one does, thus increasing dryness and potential eyestrain (Tribley et al., 2011). Frequent blinking keeps the moisture on the ocular surfaces to prevent dryness and irritation (Turgut, 2018). Also related to dryness, if prescribed, a provider is recommended to consistently wear their glasses instead of contact lenses during the consistent use of screens. This is to reduce dryness that may be created from both the contact lenses themselves in combination with CVS (Turgut, 2018). Eye drops can also be used if needed, in accordance with medical advice. Finally, while research has been somewhat variable, some have demonstrated the utility of blue-light filtering glasses in reducing CVS-like symptoms, including eyestrain and headaches (Dabrowiecki et al., 2019; Lawrenson et al., 2017). As such, providers may explore use of these nonprescription glasses.

Summary Points

- Frequent and prolonged use of videoconferencing (or general screens) can create a range of physical and ocular health issues for providers.
- Physical strategies for self-care include limiting the amount of time in front of the screen, frequent rearrangement of one's body throughout the videoconferencing sessions, ensuring the display screen is approximately eye level, using a chair that has appropriate lumbar support

and prevents slouching, placing one's shoulders and arms in a relaxed position with elbows bent between a 90- and 120-degree angle while typing, and positioning feet firmly on the floor or footrest without letting them hang in the air.

- Ocular strategies for self-care include ensuring the screen is slightly below eye level and is approximately one arm length away from the provider's eyes, taking measures to reduce glare and reflections, ensuring the screen is clean of dust, considering the use of high-contrast modes, enacting a 20-20-20 rule to briefly rest one's eyes, monitoring one's blinking to ensure appropriate eye lubrication, and wearing prescribed glasses instead of contacts. While research has been variable, some have also suggested the use of blue-light filtering glasses to reduce ocular challenges, including eyestrain and headaches.

References

Agarwal, S., Goel, D., & Sharma, A. (2013). Evaluation of the factors which contribute to the ocular complaints in computer users. *Journal of Clinical and Diagnostic Research, 7*(2), 331–335. https://doi.org/10.7860/JCDR/2013/5150.2760.

American Optometric Association (AOA). (n.d.). Computer *vision syndrome.* Retrieved from www.aoa.org/patients-and-public/caring-for-your-vision/protecting-your-vision/computer-vision-syndrome.

Cook, C., & Burgess-Limerick, R. (2003). Guidelines for computer workstations. *Ergonomics Australia, 17*(1), 19–37.

Dabrowiecki, A., Villablobos, A., & Krupinski, E. A. (2019). Impact of blue-light filtering glasses on computer vision syndrome in radiology residents: A pilot study. *Journal of Medical Imaging, 7*(2). https://doi.org/10.1117/1.JMI.7.2.022402.

Lawrenson, J. G., Hull, C. C., & Downie, L. E. (2017). The effect of blue-light blocking spectacle lenses on visual performance, macular health and the sleep–wake cycle: A systematic review of the literature. *Ophthalmic and Physiological Optics, 37*(6), 644–654.

Maheu, M. M. (2020, June 11). Zoom fatigue: What you can do about it. Telebehavioral Health Institute. Retrieved from https://telehealth.org/blog/zoom-fatigue-what-it-is-what-you-can-do/.

Occupational Safety and Health Administration (OSHA). (n.d.). Computer workstations eTool. Retrieved from www.osha.gov/SLTC/etools/computer workstations/positions.html.

Sanaeinasab, H., Saffari, M., Valipour, F., Alipour, H. R., Sepandi, M., Al Zaben, F., & Koenig, H. G. (2018). The effectiveness of a model-based health education intervention to improve ergonomic posture in office computer workers: A randomized controlled trial. *International Archives of Occupational and Environmental Health, 91*(8), 951–962. https://doi.org/10.1007/s00420-018-1336-1.

Shikdar, A. A., & Al-Kindi, M. A. (2007). Office ergonomics: Deficiencies in computer workstation design. *International Journal of Occupational Safety and Ergonomics, 13*(2), 215–223. https://doi.org/10.1080/10803548.2007.11076722.

Sklar, J. (2020, April 24). "Zoom fatigue" is taxing the brain: Here's why that happens. *National Geographic*. Retrieved from www.nationalgeographic.com/science/2020/04/coronavirus-zoom-fatigue-is-taxing-the-brain-here-is-why-that-happens/.

Tribley, J., McClain, S., Karbasi, A., & Kaldenberg, J. (2011). Tips for computer vision syndrome relief and prevention. *Work, 39*, 85–87. https://doi.org/10.3233/WOR-2011-1183.

Turgut, B. (2018). Ocular ergonomics for the computer vision syndrome. *Journal of Eye and Vision, 1*(1:2), 1–2.

18 (Brief) Answers to Common Questions About Videoconferencing Practice

The following is a collection of common questions (with answers) related to videoconferencing. Questions are grouped into three categories: general topics, delivery of services topics, and administrative topics.

General Topics

How Do I Stay Up to Date of Changes?

Given the ever-changing nature of telepsychology models, training, research, ethics, and legality, staying up to date is of the utmost importance. To gain the widest range of knowledge, providers are recommended to pursue information from multiple sources. First, providers should seek formal trainings. Whether these occur locally, nationally, or internationally, formal CE programs can be very helpful in providing different levels of expert-led training. Such trainings can be full programs, or professional discussions (e.g., The Trust roundtable discussions) of current events and challenges in telehealth-related practices. For self-learning approaches, providers can continually read about videoconferencing (or general telepsychology) happenings through recent journal articles and books, as well as telehealth-focused news outlets (e.g., ATA, National Consortium of Telehealth Resource Centers [NCTRC], Telebehavioral Health Institute), many of which have listservs that can provide digests of information (e.g., Telebehavioral Health Institute, NCTRC). For more specific resources, please see Appendices C, D, E, F, and G.

What If I'm Concerned About a Patient Recording or Taking Screenshots of the Sessions?

While a real concern, the provider can be proactive in defining rules of the videoconferencing sessions, including the limiting of recording or taking screenshots. This can be built into the informed consent process, and emphasized throughout the sessions, if reiteration is needed. To provide further protection, many videoconferencing platforms allow the provider to lock the recording and screenshot features, disabling their use for the patient. While detailing the "rules" and deactivating these features will likely remedy the issue for many patients, unfortunately, the provider simply cannot completely prevent the possibility of a patient recording or taking a screenshot. For example, while locked through the videoconferencing platform, a patient can use a third-party screen-capture program that can record their entire desktop view, including the videoconferencing window. Further, patients can take a print screen (i.e., screenshot) of their desktop, again including the videoconferencing window. Although a concern, it should be noted that this is not necessarily vastly different from F2F care in that a provider cannot always be assured that a patient is not recording the sessions through a smartphone or audio recorder in their pocket, bag, or purse.

Delivery of Services Topics

How Do I Normalize Videoconferencing for Children?

Similar to F2F services, providers should take care to normalize the use of therapeutic services for children. In the case of videoconferencing, the provider should not only normalize the therapeutic processes, but also the use of the technology. As children are often used to seeing healthcare providers in person, both the provider and caregivers taking the time to speak to the child and explain how such services are important to helping them "feel better" and "be happier" can be very important. Children should be allowed ample time to ask any and all questions they may have at the onset of the treatment.

In addition to general discussion, which may become boring to some, use of telehealth coloring pages that showcase the use of videoconferencing technologies can also help normalize the process (see Appendix K). Pages can be colored by both the provider and the patient at their respective locations before each holding their pictures up to the video camera to share. This coloring can be either a separate activity in addition to discussion, or the guiding activity for the discussion in which both can occur simultaneously.

How Do I Engage Children in the Videoconferencing Sessions?

As with F2F services, therapeutic rapport must be built and maintained, beginning at the earliest contacts. Building rapport and engaging children can sometimes be challenging and take time, as varying by many factors including their age, developmental level, attention span, and motivation for treatment. While some older children may be able to sit near the screen and appropriately participate with little effort from the provider or caregivers, others may need more structure, motivation, and breaks. Providers may initially need to start the sessions with caregivers present to facilitate the process, slowly removing them as indicated once the child's comfort grows. To further engage the child, games and media of the child's interest can be used. For example, either as the provider and patient are working together, or to be used as the break or end of session reward for participation, the provider can pull up pictures or videos, including YouTube clips. These pictures and videos can be shown on both the provider's and patient's screen via screen sharing. Alternatively, the provider could use a shared digital whiteboard program to draw with the patient (e.g., Microsoft Whiteboard), or play online multiplayer games with them (e.g., Scrabble or Battleship app). Of note, providers should consult the caregivers prior to utilizing these approaches, as some may have limits on screen time, as well as restrictions on the types of video content and games.

How Do I Normalize Videoconferencing for Older Adults (i.e., 65+ Years)?

While some research has identified that older adults may begin with a more skeptical opinion of videoconferencing services, such work has also emphasized that they often quickly warm to the process and ultimately enjoy the methods. Part of the skepticism comes from a lack of understanding of what the services are, how they work, and how they can often be equally effective when compared to F2F services, if conducted properly. Due to this, while the informed consent discussion will likely help dispel many myths and answer questions, the provider should take additional time at the onset of the videoconferencing services to answer any and all additional questions either not covered or not well clarified. In addition to answering questions, the provider should overtly detail that the videoconferencing sessions can be helpful, and how they will be used in efforts to foster hope. The provider can also explain that the use of videoconferencing can be viewed as a benefit, including by reducing the need for transportation, thus saving time and money. Finally, the provider can coordinate with the older adult or representative to adapt the videoconferencing sessions for visual or hearing-related challenges (e.g., enlarging of the image on the screen, using sound-enhancing headphones).

How Can I Make Group Videoconferencing Sessions Run Smoothly?

Due to multiple factors and participants, group videoconferencing sessions can sometimes be viewed as a daunting task. However, as with any videoconferencing consideration, a provider can create structure and guidance for group members to foster a smooth and effective meeting. To accomplish this, in addition to detailing the group processes and safety throughout the informed consent (e.g., ensuring a private location to protect confidentiality for both the individual and other group members, remaining respectful, not belittling others), the provider should supplement such information with concrete rules for how to communicate during the group. This is especially important, as different screen sizes and views may not always allow users to equally see the nonverbal behaviors that can indicate a member's intent to speak. As such, the provider may wish to enact a "three-second rule" of waiting before speaking to avoid members talking over each other and potentially not hearing information. The provider could also create a rule that if someone wants to talk, they can physically raise their hand, put a finger up, or use the platform's "raise hand" features, if available. In this way, communication and identified speakers are facilitated by the provider. While this reduces spontaneity, and such levels of control may not be desirable for some groups, it may be useful for others.

As sometimes group-member conduct may become a detriment to the group's processes (e.g., overtly rude or hostile, monopolizing), the provider should likely address such issues as they occur. An informal resolution may be sending the user a private message to adjust their behavior, or could be spoken aloud as a means of addressing the issue within the larger group, if the provider believes it is related and can be beneficial for the process. Should an individual's disruption persist as a severe detriment to the group, the provider can consider the use of a "boot" feature that is common to many platforms. This feature, although a last resort option, allows the provider who is hosting the meeting to manually remove members from the videoconferencing call. The provider can then follow up with the member after the group has concluded. Regardless of method, such processes should be detailed in the informed consent and group rules discussions, so all members are equally aware.

How Do I Conduct Mental Status Examinations Through Videoconferencing?

While predominantly possible, conducting mental status examinations through videoconferencing may require more overt effort from the provider for specific aspects of one's mental or physical health when compared to F2F interactions. For example, while affect and sensorium can be evaluated in a way similar to F2F methods, if the patient presents as sitting at the onset of the session, a provider may not get a sense of their physical mobility and gait that may come from walking the patient to the session room from a waiting area. Additionally, a provider must question the reasons for some observed potential issues, such as if the patient is speaking excessively loudly. Is this due to them having speech-volume control issues, the provider's audio settings being miscalibrated, the patient purposefully speaking loudly due to being unaware that they do not have to for the videoconferencing, or simply the patient speaking too closely to the microphone? Adapting one's evaluation for videoconferencing can include instructing a patient to stand and walk in front of the camera to evaluate gait and mobility, and directly asking about speech volumes with attempts to remedy if merely a technical-related issue.

Although predominantly possible, there are some aspects of one's mental and physical status that simply cannot be easily evaluated through videoconferencing. One of the most pertinent components is the provider's inability to smell the patient. Some providers rely on smell to identify if a patient has been using alcohol, if they have used tobacco products, or if they have exhibited poor hygiene due to their identified psychological or physical diagnoses. While creating challenges, alternative methods are possible to gather such information. For instance, related to alcohol use, providers may require that for patients to receive substance-related treatments with them, they must have a digital breathalyzer that is completed in real time on video as part of their treatment. Further, family members or friends may be able to provide collateral information regarding one's substance use or hygiene habits, although trustworthiness may be a concern for some. Alternatively, for providers who work at locations that utilize routine tests for either physical health (e.g., eating disorder-related) or substance use, the provider could mandate that for treatment to continue, patients must be evaluated for these factors at specific times through local clinics, with findings being sent directly from the clinic to the provider. While more invasive and potentially more costly for patients, some treatments may require such approaches to effectively be implemented.

How Do I Help Patients Set Up Their Videoconferencing Process?

As there are multiple aspects of setting up a proper videoconferencing process, it can sometimes be challenging for a patient to remember everything they discussed with the provider. As such, in addition to reviewing the basics of videoconferencing services through the informed consent process and discussions, the provider can supply active coaching via phone or email. As patients may become overwhelmed with too many details, the coaching can focus on the most necessary points (i.e., need for high-definition equipment, high-speed/broadband internet, antimalware programs, a private and quiet room), with additional considerations (e.g., need to avoid specific clothing that can be distracting) being addressed at a later date or as they arise. To assist providers, please see Appendix L for a handout that can be provided to patients to help them prepare for the videoconferencing sessions.

Administrative Topics

Does My Malpractice Insurance Cover Videoconferencing Sessions?

Unfortunately, due to rapid changes in the field of telehealth coverage, there is not necessarily a simple answer. The short answer to this is that some do, and some do not. As such, it would be wise for the provider to contact their malpractice insurance to ask directly, and to gain the information in writing. However, even if a provider's malpractice insurance covers their general videoconferencing practice, they may want to inquire if it covers their supervision of trainees who may be providing videoconferencing services, if applicable. Finally, beyond one's general malpractice insurance, some may consider adding cyber-liability insurance. While varying by company and policy, this relatively newer type of insurance is designed to help with cyber-based security issues including data breaches, security issues, cybercrime, or hacking to help cover legal fees, damaged networks, and hardware/software issues.

19 Conclusion and Next Steps for Providers

As based on available literature, consensus suggests that videoconferencing can be completed in an ethical, legally responsible, safe, and effective manner if both clinical and technological considerations are evaluated and integrated. To assist providers in the process, this book has provided a foundational discussion of considerations that providers can evaluate when beginning or continuing videoconferencing care. Although common factors are discussed, and the provided information can be considered a basis for one's work, providers must tailor their videoconferencing practices to meet their clinical needs, while maintaining the integrity of the psychological practices, both clinical and administrative.

Next Steps for Providers

The Need for Continued Education

Although the provided information is believed to assist one's clinical practice, it should be emphasized that this book is meant to be a beginning step, and not an end point. As with any new or developing competency, providers are encouraged to seek out additional education to ensure proper practice and expertise. This is especially important due to the high potential for novel technology-based challenges arising, for which a provider had not previously been responsible for. Telepsychology-related documentation (Appendices C, D, E), readings from peer-reviewed journal articles and books (Appendix F), and CE programming (Appendix G) can be invaluable resources to facilitate the ongoing gathering of knowledge. To supplement the educational outlets, it is suggested that providers seek informal or formal supervision and/or consultation to further guide their videoconferencing practices. Such training relationships can be helpful in relation to both the actual clinical work, as well as to the modification of one's documentation and administrative practices to account for the technology-related changes (e.g., security, scheduling, informed consent documents, billing practices).

Ongoing Assessment

In supplement of educational activities, providers should enact ongoing assessments, which can determine the strengths and areas for improvement of a provider's practice. Such assessments can focus on three specific targets. First, throughout the therapeutic services, the providers can self-reflect to review their attitudes towards the use of the technology, including any changes; their ability to provide clinical care as desired; administrative tasks; and self-care. Second, the patients can be monitored throughout their care for rupture markers, fatigue, changes in attitudes towards treatment or the technology, and general issues. Finally, as with any clinical process, general standardized outcome measures should be utilized to evaluate symptom reduction, as well as satisfaction with the services. While there are a multitude of empirically supported symptom inventories to monitor diagnostic factors, there are, with a few exceptions (e.g., Questionnaire for Assessing Patient Satisfaction with Video Teleconsultation, Fatehi et al., 2015; Telehealth Satisfaction Scale, Morgan et al., 2015; Telehealth Usability Questionnaire, Parmanto et al., 2016; Telemedicine Satisfaction Questionnaire, Yip et al., 2003), not many empirically tested telehealth satisfaction measures. Due to this, providers will likely have to adapt or create their own tailored measures. Although the items may vary from provider to provider, Table 19.1 lists possible items to consider including.

Table 19.1 Sample items for a telehealth satisfaction survey*+

- Overall, I am [satisfied/dissatisfied] with the videoconferencing services I received.
- I [enjoyed/disliked] the use of videoconferencing in my assessment/treatment.
- I believe the videoconferencing was an [effective/ineffective] means of assessment/treatment.
- I felt that the videoconferencing was [more effective/as effective/less effective] than what I would have received face-to-face.
- My videoconferencing experience was [better than/equal to/worse than] other face-to-face healthcare visits I've had.
- My favorite part of the videoconferencing services was _____.
- My least favorite part of the videoconferencing services was _____.
- I believe that _____ could be improved.
- The use of videoconferencing [made me/did not make me] feel nervous or anxious.
- If I were to seek future assessment/treatment, I would [use/avoid] videoconferencing.
- I [would/would not] recommend videoconferencing services to others.
- I felt I was [able/unable] to effectively communicate with my provider through videoconferencing without major issues.
- I felt my provider was [able/unable] to effectively understand me through videoconferencing without major issues.
- I believe that I was [able/unable] to develop a strong therapeutic relationship with my provider.
- The lack of face-to-face contact [was/was not] an issue for me.

Table 19.1 Cont.

- I felt that the videoconferencing itself [was/was not] a distraction for my assessment/treatment.
- My provider did a [great/okay/poor] job of explaining the videoconferencing assessment/treatment process before we began.
- My provider did a [great/okay/poor] job of explaining the ways to problem-solve the videoconferencing equipment if there were issues.
- I believe setting up the videoconferencing equipment (e.g., camera) was [easy/hard].
- The videoconferencing program that connected me to my provider [was/was not] easy to use.
- I was [confident/not confident] that my provider was able to help me fix any technical/equipment issues that I had.
- If there were issues with the videoconferencing, it was [easy/difficult] to get in touch with my provider.
- Overall, I was [satisfied/unsatisfied] with the video picture quality during the videoconferencing.
- Overall, I was [satisfied/unsatisfied] with the audio quality during the videoconferencing.
- Throughout my videoconferencing assessment/treatment, I experienced [a lot/some/a few/no] technical difficulties.
- The most frequent technical issues I had were _____.
- I [did/did not] take the videoconferencing assessment/treatment as seriously as I would have with face-to-face visits.
- I generally found the use of videoconferencing to be [convenient/inconvenient].
- I [did/did not] feel that the use of videoconferencing made my assessment/treatment easier to attend than if I had face-to-face visits.
- I [did/did not] feel that the use of videoconferencing was more cost effective (e.g., transportation, gas, parking, babysitter fees) than if I had face-to-face visits.
- I [did/did not] feel that the use of videoconferencing services helped save me time in my daily life.
- The use of videoconferencing made me [more/less] likely to cancel or reschedule my appointments.
- I [felt/did not feel] that the videoconferencing was a secure and private way of communicating with my provider.
- I found myself telling my provider [more/the same amount/less] about myself through the videoconferencing than I would have face-to-face.
- I found that the videoconferencing [created/did not create] eyestrain or other eye issues for me.

Notes: * Each item can be followed by a query (e.g., "What contributed to your answer?")
+ Items can be modified for Likert scale.

Conclusion

Ultimately, videoconferencing proposes a relatively unobtrusive and pre-dominantly readily available means of reaching many individuals who may otherwise go without proper services. It also allows for specialized care to be provided where it was previously unavailable. While a provider must consider multiple components to ensure proper usage, videoconferencing has the potential to positively impact one's practice, patient care, and society at large.

References

Fatehi, F., Martin-Khan, M., Smith, A. C., Russell, A. W., & Gray, L. C. (2015). Patient satisfaction with video teleconsultation in a virtual diabetes outreach clinic. *Diabetes Technology & Therapeutics, 17*(1), 43–48. https://doi.org/10.1089/dia.2014.0159.

Morgan, D. G., Kosteniuk, J., Stewart, N., O'Connell, M. E., Karunanyake, C., & Beever, R. (2015). The Telehealth Satisfaction Scale (TeSS): Reliability, validity, and satisfaction with telehealth in a rural memory clinic population. *Telemedicine and e-Health, 20*(11), 997–1003. https://doi.org/10.1089/tmj.2014.0002.

Parmanto, B., Lewis, A. N., Jr., Graham, K. M., & Bertolet, M. H. (2016). Development of the Telehealth Usability Questionnaire (TUQ). *International Journal of Telerehabilitation, 8*(1), 3–10. https://doi.org/10.5195/ijt.2016.6196.

Yip, M. P., Chang, A. M., Chan, J., & Mackenzie, A. E. (2003). Development of the Telemedicine Satisfaction Questionnaire to evaluate patient satisfaction with telemedicine: A preliminary study. *Journal of Telemedicine and Telecare, 9*(1), 45–50. https://doi.org/10.1258/135763303321159693.

Appendix A: Acronyms Used in This Book

American Counseling Association	ACA
American Medical Association	AMA
American Optometric Association	AOA
American Psychological Association	APA
American Telemedicine Association	ATA
Association of Social Work Boards	ASWB
Association of State and Provincial Psychology Boards	ASPPB
attention-deficit/hyperactivity disorder	ADHD
Authority to Practice Interjurisdictional Telepsychology	APIT
business associations agreement	BAA
Canadian Psychological Association	CPA
central processing unit	CPU
Children's Online Privacy Protection Act	COPPA
Clinical Social Work Association	CSWA
cognitive behavioral therapy	CBT
computer vision syndrome	CVS
continuing education	CE
Council on Social Work Education	CSWE
electronic health record	EHR
electronic-protected health information	e-PHI
Examination for Professional Practice in Psychology	EPPP
face to face	F2F
Family Education Rights and Privacy Act	FERPA
Federal Communications Commission	FCC
General Data Protection Regulation	GDPR
Health Information Technology for Economic and Clinical Health	HITECH
Health Insurance Portability and Accountability Act	HIPAA

Health Resources and Services Administration	HRSA
Military Health System	MHS
National Association of Social Workers	NASW
National Consortium of Telehealth Resource Centers	NCTRC
National Cybersecurity Center of Excellence	NCCoE
National Institute of Mental Health	NIMH
National Institute of Standards and Technology	NIST
obsessive-compulsive disorder	OCD
Occupational Safety and Health Administration	OSHA
operating system	OS
pan–tilt–zoom	PTZ
Personal Information Protection and Electronic Document Act	PIPEDA
picture-in-picture	PIP
protected health information	PHI
Psychological Interjurisdictional Compact	PSYPACT
random access memory	RAM
round-trip time	RTT
socioeconomic status	SES
US Department of Health and Human Services	HHS
US Department of Veterans Affairs	VA
World Health Organization	WHO

Appendix B: Helpful Videoconferencing-Specific Definitions

Asynchronous Services

- Information is collected and transmitted at another time to another location (i.e., not live; e.g., email). This type of service is often referred to as "store-and-forward."

Bandwidth

- Maximum rate of data transfer per second over an internet connection.

Broadband Internet

- A form of "always on" high-speed internet access that encompasses several types of technologies including fiber optics, wireless, cable, satellite, and DSL.

Business Associate

- In a business associate's agreement, the business associate is a person or organization other than a member of the covered entity who performs functions or activities on behalf of the covered entity and has access to PHI or e-PHI.

Business Associate's Agreement (BAA)

- A contract between a covered entity and the business associate that serves as an agreement that the business associate will protect any PHI or e-PHI they come into contact with. A BAA helps protect the provider and their practice from liability in the event of a data breach associated with the business associate vendor.

Central Process Unit (CPU)

- One of the main components in making a computer run. It is a piece of hardware that allows a computer to interact with applications and programs to translate the data and create output that is presented on the user's display screen.

Compression

- Allows for images and video to consume less space.

Covered Entity

- In a business associate's agreement, the covered entity is the provider or provider's organization.

Decryption

- The process of returning encrypted data to a readable and understandable state.

Distant Site

- The site of the provider, sometimes referred to as the "hub." The distant site may be a clinic, community center, or residence from which the provider is supplying services.

Effectiveness

- Extent to which an intervention produces beneficial outcomes under ordinary day-to-day circumstances (i.e., real life without research-based controls).

Efficacy

- Extent to which an intervention can produce a beneficial outcome under ideal circumstances (i.e., experimental controls).

Encryption

- A method of converting regular text and data into encoded information, making the information unreadable to unauthorized individuals without a deciphering key to decrypt the data.

Firewall

- Network security that controls data coming in and out of one's computer system as based upon set rules (i.e., communication between trusted and untrusted networks).

Hardware (Computer System)

- The physical parts of a computer system, including the CPU, RAM, graphic cards, sound card, mouse, and keyboard.

Hybrid Services

- Combination of synchronous and asynchronous, and/or in-person services.

Informed Consent

- Providing a patient with information regarding all aspects of the service relationship (e.g., benefits, limitations, patient role, provider role, billing practices, alternatives to proposed treatment) so that the patient can make an informed decision about whether to pursue the proposed services or seek alternatives.

Interjurisdictional Compact

- A legal agreement between states that sign the compact into law. If a provider is accepted into the compact, they will be able to practice without an additional license in any state that has ratified the compact into law.

Jitter

- Inconsistency in the latency (i.e., delays) of packets going between two network points.

Jurisdiction

- The geographic area of which an authority, such as a court, extends.

Latency

- The time required for a signal to travel from a source to a destination (i.e., delay).

Malware

- Broadly defined as computer software designed to cause damage or make a computer system susceptible to others (e.g., virus, ransomware).

mHealth

- Mobile health – the use of mobile technology (e.g., smartphones, apps) in healthcare services.

Originating Site

- The site of the patient, sometimes referred to as the "spoke." The originating site may be a clinic, community center, or residence where the patient is receiving services.

Packet

- Formatted data units.

Packet Loss

- Discarded packet information. The higher the amount of packet loss, the more video or audio issues that can occur, including on-screen artifacts.

Pixel

- Tiny squares that make up a digital image.

Psychological Interjurisdictional Compact (PSYPACT)

- Clinical psychology-specific interjurisdictional compact.

Random Access Memory (RAM):

- Computer hardware that allows a computer to temporarily store short-term or working data.

Resolution

- How many pixels an image contains, determining how clear the image quality looks to the user.

Software (Computer System)

- Programs or code installed onto and used by a computer system.

Synchronous Services

- Live, real-time communication, often between a patient and provider.

System

- The full computer, tablet, smartphone or other technology.

Telehealth

- Umbrella term for the integration of technology in health services.

Telepresence

- Also referred to as eye-gaze angle, telepresence is the angle between the eye and the camera, and the eye and the center of the display screen. This process involves placement of the patient's image so that their head and eyes are in close proximity to the provider's video camera. In doing so, by looking at the video image, it appears as though the provider is looking into the camera and thus making direct eye contact with the patient.

Telemedicine

- Technology use and integration for medical healthcare.

Telepsychology

- Technology use and integration for psychological/mental healthcare.

Appendix C: Consolidated Mental Health Resources

Formal Guidelines and Recommendations from Guiding Organizations

Please note that all information is for resource purposes only, with copyrights reserved by their respective owners.

Organization	Resource	Weblink
American Counseling Association	*Ethical and Professional Standards*	www.counseling.org/knowledge-center/ethics#2014code
American Psychological Association	*Guidelines for the Practice of Telepsychology*	www.apa.org/practice/guidelines/telepsychology
American Telemedicine Association	*ATA Practice Guidelines for Video-Based Online Mental Health Services*	www.liebertpub.com/doi/abs/10.1089/tmj.2013.9989 or www.americantelemed.org/resources/practice-guidelines-for-video-based-online-mental-health-services-2/
American Telemedicine Association	*Utilization of the American Telemedicine Association's Clinical Practice Guidelines*	www.liebertpub.com/doi/10.1089/tmj.2013.0027
American Telemedicine Association	*American Telemedicine Association Practice Guidelines for Telemental Health with Children and Adolescents*	www.liebertpub.com/doi/10.1089/tmj.2017.0177 or www.americantelemed.org/resources/practice-guidelines-for-telemental-health-with-children-and-adolescents/
American Telemedicine Association	*Operating Procedures for Pediatric Telehealth*	https://pediatrics.aappublications.org/content/pediatrics/140/2/e20171756.full.pdf or www.americantelemed.org/resources/operating-procedures-for-pediatric-telehealth/

Organization	Resource	Weblink
American Telemedicine Association	*A Concise Guide for Telemedicine Practitioners: Human Factors Quick Guide Eye Contact*	www.americantelemed.org/resources/a-concise-guide-for-telemedicine-practitioners-human-factors-quick-guide-eye-contact/
American Telemedicine Association	*Let There Be Light: A Quick Guide to Telemedicine Lighting*	www.americantelemed.org/resources/let-there-be-light-a-quick-guide-to-telemedicine-lighting/
American Telemedicine Association	*Evidence-Based Practice for Telemental Health*	www.americantelemed.org/resources/evidence-based-practice-for-telemental-health/
American Telemedicine Association	*Practice Guidelines for Videoconferencing Telemental Health*	www.americantelemed.org/resources/practice-guidelines-for-videoconferencing-telemental-health/
American Telemedicine Association	*Home Telehealth Clinical Guidelines*	www.americantelemed.org/resources/home-telehealth-clinical-guidelines/
National Association of Social Workers, Association of Social Work Boards, Council on Social Work Education, Clinical Social Work Association	*Technology in Social Work Practice*	www.socialworkers.org/includes/newIncludes/homepage/PRA-BRO-33617.TechStandards_FINAL_POSTING.pdf
National Association of School Psychologists	*Guidance for Delivery of School Psychological Telehealth Services*	www.nasponline.org/assets/documents/Guidance_Telehealth_Virtual_Service_%20Delivery_Final%20(2).pdf
National Association of School Psychologists	*Telehealth: Virtual Service Delivery Updated Recommendations*	www.nasponline.org/resources-and-publications/resources-and-podcasts/covid-19-resource-center/special-education-resources/telehealth-virtual-service-delivery-updated-recommendations

Appendix D: Consolidated Mental Health Resources

Helpful Documents, Websites, and Toolkits

Please note that all information is for resource purposes only, with copyrights reserved by their respective owners.

Organization	Resource	Weblink
American Academy of Pediatrics	*Getting Started in Telehealth*	www.aap.org/en-us/professional-resources/practice-transformation/telehealth/Pages/Getting-Started-in-Telehealth.aspx
American Counseling Association	*Telebehavioral Health Information and Counselors in Health Care*	www.counseling.org/knowledge-center/mental-health-resources/trauma-disaster/telehealth-information-and-counselors-in-health-care
American Psychiatric Association	*Telepsychiatry Practice Guidelines Toolkit*	www.psychiatry.org/psychiatrists/practice/telepsychiatry/toolkit/practice-guidelines
American Psychological Association	*Office and Technology Checklist for Telepsychological Services*	www.apa.org/practice/programs/dmhi/research-information/telepsychological-services-checklist
Association of State and Provincial Psychology Boards	*PSYPACT – Psychology Interjurisdictional Compact*	www.asppb.net/mpage/legislative
Center for Connected Health Policy	*Current State Laws and Reimbursement Policies*	www.cchpca.org/telehealth-policy/current-state-laws-and-reimbursement-policies#
Epstein, Becker, and Green	*Telemental Health Laws*	www.ebglaw.com/telemental-health-laws-app/
Helping Give Away Psychological Science/ Telepsychology	*Guidelines for Conducting Mental Health Services with Technology*	https://en.wikiversity.org/wiki/Helping_Give_Away_Psychological_Science/Telepsychology

Organization	Resource	Weblink
National Association of Social Workers	*Clinical Social Work Practice Tools: Technology*	www.socialworkers.org/Practice/ Clinical-Social-Work/Technology
National Consortium of Telehealth Resource Centers	*Telehealth Etiquette Checklist*	www.telehealthresourcecenter.org/ wp-content/uploads/2019/07/ Telehealth-Etiquette-Checklist. pdf
Pearson	*Staying Connected Through Telepractice*	www.pearsonassessments.com/ professional-assessments/digital-solutions/telepractice/products. html
Telebehavioral Health Institute	*Telebehavioral Health Institute's Buyer's Guide*	https://telehealth.org/buyersguide/
TelehealthROCKS – University of Kansas Medical Center	*Rural Outreach for the Children of Kansas*	www.telehealthrocks.org/

Appendix E: Consolidated Mental Health Resources

Helpful Organizations

Organization	Weblink
American Academy of Pediatrics	www.aap.org/en-us/Pages/Default.aspx
American Counseling Association	www.counseling.org/
American Medical Association	www.ama-assn.org/
American Psychiatric Association	www.psychiatry.org/
American Psychological Association	www.apa.org/
American Telemedicine Association	www.americantelemed.org/
Center for Connected Health Policy	www.cchpca.org/
National Association of School Psychologists	www.nasponline.org/
National Association of Social Workers	www.socialworkers.org/
National Consortium of Telehealth Resource Centers	www.telehealthresourcecenter.org/
Person Centered Tech	https://personcenteredtech.com/
National Telehealth Technology Assessment Resource Center	http://telehealthtechnology.org/
Telebehavioral Health Institute	https://telehealth.org/

Appendix F: Helpful Journals and Books

Journal name	Weblink
Australian Psychologist	https://aps.onlinelibrary.wiley.com/journal/17429544
Clinical Psychology: Research and Practice	https://onlinelibrary.wiley.com/journal/14682850
Computers in Human Behavior	www.journals.elsevier.com/computers-in-human-behavior
Cyberpsychology, Behavior, and Social Networking	www.liebertpub.com/loi/cyber
International Journal of Telemedicine and Applications	www.hindawi.com/journals/ijta/
International Journal of Technology Assessment in Health Care	www.cambridge.org/core/journals/international-journal-of-technology-assessment-in-health-care
Internet Interventions	www.journals.elsevier.com/internet-interventions
JMIR Mental Health	https://mental.jmir.org/
JMIR mHealth and uHealth	https://mhealth.jmir.org/
Journal of Clinical Psychology	https://onlinelibrary.wiley.com/journal/10974679
Journal of Medical Internet Research	www.jmir.org/
Journal of Technology in Behavioral Science	www.springer.com/journal/41347
Journal of Technology in Human Services	www.tandfonline.com/toc/wths20/current
Journal of the American Medical Association	https://jamanetwork.com/
Journal of Telemedicine and Telecare	https://journals.sagepub.com/home/jtt
Professional Psychology: Research and Practice	www.apa.org/pubs/journals/pro/

Journal name	Weblink
Psychological Services	www.apa.org/pubs/journals/ser/
Psychiatric Services	https://ps.psychiatryonline.org/
Rural and Remote Health	www.rrh.org.au/
Telemedicine and e-Health	https://home.liebertpub.com/ publications/telemedicine-and-e-health/54

Appendix G: Continuing Education Programming

Organization	Weblink
American Counseling Association	www.counseling.org/continuing-education
American Psychological Association	www.apa.org/education/ce/topic/?query=cetopic:Telehealth
American Telemedicine Association	www.americantelemed.org/resource/recorded-content/
National Register of Health Service Psychologists	https://ce.nationalregister.org/
Person Centered Tech	https://personcenteredtech.com/
PESI	www.pesi.com/
Telebehavioral Health Institute	https://telehealth.org/
Telehealth Certification Institute	https://telementalhealthtraining.com/
Trust Parma	https://parma.trustinsurance.com/Workshops-Webinars
Zur Institute	www.zurinstitute.com/

Appendix H: Summary Overview of Processes for the Utilization of Videoconferencing

Topic	Brief summary of process
Evaluate the research base to ensure knowledge	• A provider should critically review the literature base to determine under which circumstances videoconferencing has been demonstrated as efficacious or effective (e.g., age, gender, diagnostic condition, setting), how services differ from F2F care, how the videoconferencing affects therapeutic alliance, how to ensure safety, means of monitoring progress, and assessment and treatment types translated to distance administration. Both benefits and limitations should be reviewed to guide practice. • Combined knowledge should contribute to how the provider conducts the videoconferencing sessions and how they problem-solve arising issues to minimize the impact on the care.
Review ethical guidelines	• A provider should review the ethical guidelines that correspond to their governing organizations. • Ethical standards relate to the provider, patient, technology, and administrative processes. • Ethical considerations include the provider reviewing research and securing proper training related to the videoconferencing services, establishing patient appropriateness, ensuring informed consent, safeguarding privacy and security, and safety planning.
Review legal guidelines of jurisdiction(s)	• A provider should review the legal regulations and laws that govern their practice in any location of their work. This includes both the provider's location of practice, and the patient's location where they receive the services. • Laws may vary by state and country (e.g., HIPAA, GDPR, PIPEDA). • Legal considerations include licensing, cross-jurisdiction practice, and acceptable reasons for breaking confidentiality.
Evaluate the systems	• Both the provider's and patient's systems should be powerful enough to manage a seamless videoconferencing session. • A provider should ensure that all systems used are secure, with proper security and antimalware software installed.

Topic	Brief summary of process
Evaluate the video cameras	• Both the provider and the patient should seek video cameras that are easy to install, have high-definition video, and are easy to problem-solve. The ability to pan, tilt, and zoom; modify resolution; and adjust compression options are also valuable features. • Common commercially available video cameras are often either built into one's pre-existing system, or are plug-and-play USB.
Evaluate the display screen options	• To complement the high-definition video camera, the provider and the patient should utilize size-appropriate high-definition screens (e.g., desktop computer monitor, laptop monitor).
Evaluate microphone options	• To supplement the high-definition video, a provider should ensure appropriate microphones for both themselves and the patient. • Microphones can be built into one's pre-existing system, built into a plug-and-play USB video camera/microphone combination, or added separately.
Evaluate the videoconferencing platform	• A videoconferencing platform should be selected that allows for high-definition video and audio, as well as security compliance (e.g., ≥128-bit encryption, signed BAA). • Factors to consider when selecting a platform include the cost (e.g., subscription costs), functions (e.g., high-definition, screen share, multiple simultaneous users), and security (e.g., encryption standards, password protections).
Evaluate the bandwidth and latency	• In order to see and hear each other in real time without any issues (e.g., freezing), the provider and the patient should evaluate both bandwidth and latency. Users should strive for at least 384 KBPS for bandwidth, and less than 150 milliseconds of one-way latency (with ≤ 30 milliseconds of jitter and ≤ 1 percent packet loss).
Evaluate the room setup	• Both the provider and patient's selected rooms for the videoconferencing should appear as close to a normal office or consulting room as possible. Both should avoid messy or distracting rooms, opting for a pleasant and neat atmosphere. • The background of the provider and patient should be uncluttered and devoid of significantly distracting objects. Background blocking devices can be used, if needed. • A provider and patient should minimize the possibility of interruptions. • A provider and patient should ensure proper lighting of a room, putting the light behind the camera and avoiding the aiming of cameras towards windows, reflective surfaces, hallways, or doors that can create distractions.

Topic	Brief summary of process
Evaluate the session's video quality	• The provider and patient should avoid brightly pattered, striped, checkered, or reflective clothing. • The provider and patient should avoid bright whites, reds, or orange clothing. • The provider and patient should avoid dangling jewelry. • The provider and patient should conduct an explicit video test for both ends at the onset of each session. • The provider and patient should turn off the PIP feature of the videoconferencing platform, if possible. • The provider and patient should have the other's image in a location near the camera to foster telepresence. • At the end of the session, the provider should turn off their video camera.
Evaluate the session's audio quality	• The provider and patient should avoid noise-making clothing and jewelry. • The provider and patient should conduct an explicit sound test for both ends at the onset of each session. • The provider and patient should turn off all distractions at the onset of the session (e.g., pop-up reminders, phone ringers). • The provider and patient should avoid making noises that may be amplified during the session (e.g., typing, rustling with papers, writing on hard surfaces). • At the end of the session, the provider should mute the microphone.
Document	• A provider should document both the clinical and videoconferencing-specific factors of a session. • General documentation can include a rationale for the videoconferencing being rendered in replacement of F2F, platforms used, if issues were encountered with the technology and how they were resolved, an indication of the provider's location (i.e., distant site), an indication of the patient's location (i.e., originating site), a statement of verification of the patient's identity, and emergency contact information. • For an initial contact note, additional information a provider should consider incorporating includes the evaluation procedures to ensure patient appropriateness for the videoconferencing, the informed consent process, and if a safety code word or phrase was created. • For an assessment note, additional information a provider should consider incorporating includes indications that the patient agreed not to record the assessment process, that the patient agreed to complete the assessment independently, details on how the assessment was conducted, and a clinical statement about the validity of the data yielded from the videoconferencing assessment.

Topic	Brief summary of process
Self-care	• Given the potential for increased physical and ocular challenges as a result of increased technology use, a provider should enact self-care techniques including taking breaks, frequent rearrangement of one's body during sessions, adjusting the monitor's level to approximately eye level, using appropriate chairs that provide lumbar support, reducing glare or dust, and monitoring one's blinking to avoid eyestrain and dry eyes.
Be knowledgeable of available resources	• A provider should be aware of resources to help guide their practice. Resources may include guidebooks from guiding organizations, up-to-date literature, up-to-date websites, and colleague support (e.g., listserv discussions, organization members).

Appendix I: Comprehensive Videoconferencing Provider Checklist

Component	Description	Done?
Pre-videoconferencing activities		
1. Completed training	Received videoconferencing-specific training and/or completed CE programming.	☐
2. Evaluated the research base	Reviewed up-to-date research, books, and documentation regarding videoconferencing practice.	☐
	Evaluated relevant research for settings/location to be used.	☐
	Evaluated relevant research for ages and genders to be treated.	☐
	Evaluated relevant research for psychological condition(s) to be treated.	☐
	Evaluated relevant research for assessment and/or intervention approaches to be utilized.	☐
3. Reviewed ethical guidelines	Read relevant ethics-related practice guidelines from guiding organizations.	☐
	Knowledgeable of benefits of videoconferencing services.	☐
	Knowledgeable of limitations of videoconferencing services.	☐
	Knowledgeable of differences of videoconferencing services as compared to F2F.	☐
	Knowledgeable on ethical considerations of confidentiality as unique to videoconferencing services.	☐
	Knowledgeable of safety planning related to videoconferencing services.	☐

Component	Description	Done?
4. Reviewed legal guidelines	Knowledgeable of state and national (or country) laws relevant to general clinical services.	☐
	Knowledgeable of state and national (or country) laws relevant to technology use in clinical services.	☐
	Knowledgeable of laws related to involuntary hospitalization in all locations of practice.	☐
	Licensed in all jurisdictions of practice, or entered into interjurisdictional compact for all states of service provision.	☐
5. Evaluated patient appropriateness	Evaluated patient's general feelings towards mental health services.	☐
	Evaluated patient's general feelings and comfort towards technology.	☐
	Evaluated if patient has attempted psychological services in past, and outcomes (e.g., positive experience, helpful, would do again).	☐
	Evaluated if patient has attempted telepsychology-based services in the past, and outcomes (e.g., positive experience, helpful, would do again).	☐
	Evaluated patient's feelings about specifically receiving videoconferencing.	☐
	Evaluated if patient has any cognitive or sensory issues that may create challenges for videoconferencing.	☐
	Evaluated if patient has a high-risk mental health diagnosis.	☐
	Evaluated if patient has suicidal ideation, plan, or intent.	☐
	Evaluated if patient has homicidal ideation, plan, or intent.	☐
	Evaluated if patient has access to firearms or other weapons (e.g., knives, machinery).	☐
	Evaluated if patient is actively using alcohol or other legal substances.	☐
	Evaluated if patient is actively using illicit substances.	☐
	Evaluated patient's need for technical aids (e.g., headsets).	☐
	Evaluated potential for patient to experience fatigue or discomfort from use of technology.	☐
	Evaluated if patient has an appropriate, private area for the videoconferencing.	☐
	Evaluated if patient has reasonable hardware and software to run videoconferencing.	☐

Component	Description	Done?
	Evaluated rationale for videoconferencing usage (e.g., patient's distance from the provider's practice, transportation issues, time limitations, availability of general or specialist F2F services in their area).	☐
	Evaluated if patient has support systems to assist if needed (e.g., family, friends).	☐
	Evaluated location of nearest medical center, in case of emergency.	☐
	Evaluated location of nearest law enforcement center, in case of emergency.	☐
6. Conducted informed consent	Adapted F2F informed consent processes, or created videoconferencing-specific informed consent processes.	☐
	Detailed informed consent information in writing and documented in medical record.	☐
	Detailed informed consent information verbally and documented the discussion.	☐
	(Informed consent form and discussion) Indication of standard practice – types of therapy provided.	☐
	(Informed consent form and discussion) Indication of standard practice – acceptable videoconferencing platforms.	☐
	(Informed consent form and discussion) Indication of standard practice – indication that patient agreed to only receive services in pre-approved locations (e.g., physical area, state provider is licensed in).	☐
	(Informed consent form and discussion) Indication of standard practice – indication if trainees will participate.	☐
	(Informed consent form and discussion) Strengths and limitations – indication of videoconferencing research as an emerging field.	☐
	(Informed consent form and discussion) Strengths and limitations – indication of current outcome data.	☐
	(Informed consent form and discussion) Strengths and limitations – detailing of benefits including potential convenience, the potential for improved access to care and less wait, the potential for overcoming disabilities, and the potential for economic benefits associated with decreased transportation costs.	☐

Component	Description	Done?
	(Informed consent form and discussion) Strengths and limitations – detailing of limitations including the potential for interruptions and reduced confidentiality, the potential for technology-related challenges (e.g., latency issues, video/audio issues, drop in video call), the potential for eyestrain, the potential for a reduced ability to see nonverbal behaviors, the potential costs of securing technology, the lack of a "cool-down" period after sessions end, and ongoing legal changes.	☐
	(Informed consent form and discussion) General delivery factors – discussion of similarities to F2F care.	☐
	(Informed consent form and discussion) General delivery factors – discussion of differences to F2F care.	☐
	(Informed consent form and discussion) General delivery factors – discussion of minimal hardware and software specifications for videoconferencing.	☐
	(Informed consent form and discussion) General delivery factors – discussion of management of crises.	☐
	(Informed consent form and discussion) General delivery factors – discussion of what will be included in the medical record related to the videoconferencing sessions (e.g., between session emails).	☐
	(Informed consent form and discussion) Communication – discussed between-session contact methods.	☐
	(Informed consent form and discussion) Communication – discussed hours of provider work.	☐
	(Informed consent form and discussion) Communication – discussed average communication response time.	☐
	(Informed consent form and discussion) Communication – discussed information to communicate to the provider versus immediately going to a hospital.	☐
	(Informed consent form and discussion) Troubleshooting – discussed methods of troubleshooting issues that may arise (e.g., latency/freezing, internet disconnections, audio/video issues).	☐
	(Informed consent form and discussion) Troubleshooting – discussed options (e.g., telephone, reschedule session) should videoconferencing not be viable.	☐

Component	Description	Done?
	(Informed consent form and discussion) Administrative – discussed fees and billing.	☐
	(Informed consent form and discussion) Administrative – discussed ways to schedule appointments.	☐
	(Informed consent form and discussion) Administrative – discussed attendance expectations.	☐
	Secured patient's signed agreement.	☐
7. Gathered emergency contacts	Name of patient.	☐
	Address of patient while receiving videoconferencing services.	☐
	Description of location where patient will receive videoconferencing services.	☐
	Phone number of patient.	☐
	Email of patient.	☐
	Alternative contact – name.	☐
	Alternative contact – relationship to patient.	☐
	Alternative contact – address.	☐
	Alternative contact – distance from patient.	☐
	Alternative contact – phone number.	☐
	Alternative contact – email.	☐
	Signed release of information form for provider to contact alternative individuals, if needed.	☐
	Nearest medical center – name.	☐
	Nearest medical center – address.	☐
	Nearest medical center – phone number.	☐
	Nearest law enforcement office – name.	☐
	Nearest law enforcement office – address.	☐
	Nearest law enforcement office – phone number.	☐

Component	Description	Done?
	Created step-by-step plan of managing crises.	☐
	Emergency information is in readily accessible location in medical record.	☐
	Provided copies of information to patient.	☐
8. Reviewed data security	Ensured at least 128-bit encryption for videoconferencing platform.	☐
	Ensured a signed BAA with third-party videoconferencing platform company.	☐
	Ensured physical safeguards of physical premises and hardware.	☐
	Ensured administrative safeguards including training for all staff members with access to the technology or PHI or e-PHI.	☐
	Ensured technical safeguards for systems including antimalware software, personal and network firewalls, network access control for the provider, use of passwords, and use of at least 128-bit encryption.	☐
9. Created data breach plan	Designed a protocol to conduct a risk assessment, provide notice to patients affected, and provide notice to DHHS.	☐
Videoconferencing considerations		
10. Considered systems	Evaluated and tested provider's system to ensure smooth and high-definition videoconferencing.	☐
	Evaluated and tested patient's systems to ensure smooth and high-definition videoconferencing.	☐
	Ensured appropriate antimalware software on provider's system.	☐
	Ensured appropriate antimalware software on patient's systems.	☐
11. Considered video cameras	Evaluated and tested to ensure provider's video camera is appropriate for high-definition image.	☐
	Evaluated and tested to ensure patient's video camera is appropriate for high-definition image.	☐
	Reviewed if provider's software allows for changing of video resolution and compression.	☐
	Reviewed if patient's camera (with provider software control) allows for panning, tilting, and zooming.	☐
12. Considered display screens	Ensured the provider has an appropriate screen size and quality to complement the video camera.	☐

Component	Description	Done?
	Ensured the patient has an appropriate screen size and quality to complement the video camera.	☐
13. Considered microphones	Evaluated and tested to ensure provider's microphone/audio is appropriate and clear.	☐
	Evaluated and tested to ensure patient's microphone/audio is appropriate and clear.	☐
14. Considered platforms	Evaluated and secured appropriate videoconferencing platform as based upon cost, functions, and security.	☐
15. Considered bandwidth and latency	Evaluated provider's bandwidth to ensure smooth and high-definition video and audio.	☐
	Evaluated patient's bandwidth to ensure smooth and high-definition video and audio.	☐
	Evaluated provider's latency to ensure smooth and high-definition video and audio.	☐
	Evaluated patient's latency to ensure smooth and high-definition video and audio.	☐
16. Considered room setup	Evaluated the appropriateness of the provider's videoconferencing room.	☐
	Evaluated the appropriateness of the patient's videoconferencing room.	☐
	Provider took precautions to reduce interruptions and loss of privacy.	☐
	Patient took precautions to reduce interruptions and loss of privacy.	☐
	Provider ensured that their camera placement is appropriate to view the provider, while reducing distractions or lighting issues.	☐
	Provider coached the patient to ensure that their camera placement is appropriate to view the patient, while reducing distractions or lighting issues.	☐
	Provider adjusted the patient's video image and their camera placement to simulate appropriate eye gaze (i.e., telepresence).	☐
17. Considered video	The provider avoided wearing bright, patterned, striped, checkered, or reflective clothing.	☐
	The patient avoided wearing bright, patterned, striped, checkered, or reflective clothing.	☐
	The provider avoided wearing any hanging or distracting jewelry.	☐
	The patient avoided wearing any hanging or distracting jewelry.	☐
	The provider avoided fidgeting behaviors.	☐
	The patient avoided fidgeting behaviors.	☐

Component	Description	Done?
18. Considered audio	The provider avoided any noisy clothing or jewelry.	☐
	The patient avoided any noisy clothing or jewelry.	☐
	The provider adjusted their audio volume and speaking distance from the microphone to ensure clarity.	☐
	The patient adjusted their audio volume and speaking distance from the microphone to ensure clarity.	☐

Videoconferencing implementation

Component	Description	Done?
19. Sent links and handouts	Sent the patient a link to the videoconferencing session.	☐
	Sent the patient handouts for the videoconferencing session.	☐
20. Verified information	Verified the patient's identity at the onset of the session.	☐
	Verified the patient's location at the onset of the session.	☐
	Verified the patient is in a private location at the onset of the session.	☐
	Verified appropriate video quality for provider at the onset of the session.	☐
	Verified appropriate video quality for patient at the onset of the session.	☐
	Verified appropriate audio quality for provider at the onset of the session.	☐
	Verified appropriate audio quality for patient at the onset of the session.	☐
21. Documented the session	Documented the rationale for videoconferencing being rendered in replacement of, or in supplement of, F2F care.	☐
	Documented the videoconferencing platforms used.	☐
	Documented if issues presented and how they were resolved.	☐
	Documented the provider's location.	☐
	Documented the patient's location.	☐
	Documented that identifies were verified.	☐
	Documented that the patient's location was verified.	☐
	Documented emergency contact information.	☐
	(If created) documented if safety word/phrase was used.	☐

Component	Description	Done?
	(If applicable to session content) documented patient appropriateness screening process.	☐
	(If applicable to session content) documented informed consent process.	☐
	(If applicable to session content) documented right of provider to cease videoconferencing at any time as based upon provider judgment.	☐
22. Considered self-care	Limited the amount of continuous time spent in front of screen without moving.	☐
	Took standing/walking breaks every 45–60 minutes.	☐
	Frequently adjusted body to avoid remaining in same position for extended periods.	☐
	Used chair that supplied back support and conformed to spine.	☐
	Positioned elbows at 90- to 120-degree angle for typing.	☐
	Positioned feet either firmly on floor, or on a footrest.	☐
	Positioned knees at about the same height as hips with feet slightly forward.	☐
	Positioned display screen at eye level Positioned screen at least 20–25 inches away from eyes.	☐
	Reduced glare, reflections, and dust of screen.	☐
	Increased contrast of image and fonts, as needed.	☐
	Enacted 20-20-20 rule for eyes.	☐
	Took approximately 15-minute break once every two hours of continuous screen time.	☐
	Made efforts to blink more frequently.	☐
	Utilized prescription glasses instead of contacts, if reasonable.	☐
	Considered using blue-light blocking glasses.	☐
23. Aware of resources to guide work	Aware of journals, books, websites, and other resources to help providers stay up to date and guide their continued practice.	☐

Appendix J: Simplified Videoconferencing Provider Checklist

Component	Completed?
Setting up the videoconferencing sessions	
1. Verified appropriateness of patient for videoconferencing clinical work.	☐
2. Verified appropriateness of location and environment.	☐
3. Gathered verbal and written informed consent.	☐
4. Gathered emergency contact and created safety plan.	☐
5. Verified expectations of processes and communication.	☐
6. Coached the patient to set up environments to maximize videoconferencing.	☐
7. Discussed troubleshooting and problem-solving, and created formal plan.	☐
8. Created safety word or phrase to indicate that the provider should immediately end session.	☐
Conducting the videoconferencing sessions	
1. Sent link to videoconferencing session.	☐
2. Sent handouts via a secure email platform.	☐
3. Explicitly tested video and audio equipment at the onset of the session.	☐
4. Verified identify of the patient at the onset of the session.	☐
5. Verified location of the patient at the onset of the session.	☐

Component	Completed?
6. Confirmed the patient was alone and/or participants were known to the provider.	☐
7. Verified that all nonessential programs were closed to avoid system slowing or interruptions.	☐
8. Verified that all users minimized potential interruptions (e.g., phone, email notifications).	☐
9. Conducted the clinical session as appropriate and problem-solved any issues that arose.	☐
10. Turned off the video and muted the audio at the conclusion of the session.	☐
11a. Documented the session – rationale for videoconferencing services.	☐
11b. Documented the session – platform used.	☐
11c. Documented the session – if issues arose and how they were addressed.	☐
11d. Documented the session – verified identities and location at the onset of the session.	☐

Appendix K: Videoconferencing Coloring Pages for Children

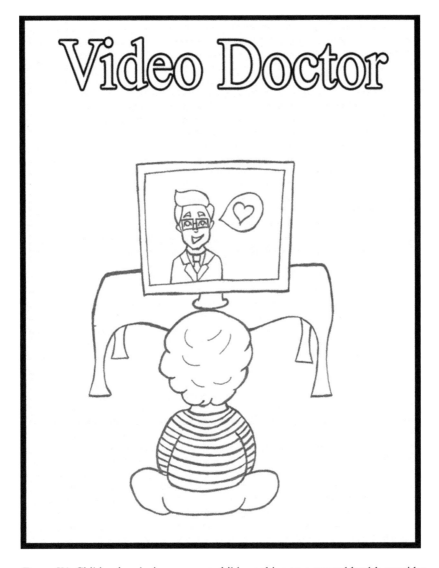

Figure K1 Children's coloring page – a child speaking to a mental health provider through videoconferencing.

Source: Perle, A. (2020). Children's coloring page - A child speaking to a mental health provider through videoconferencing [Unpubished drawing].

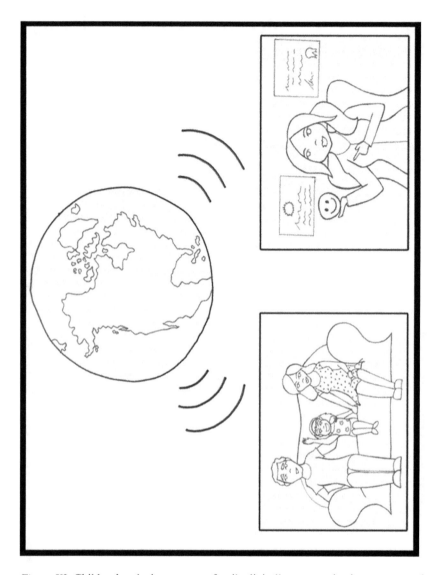

Figure K2 Children's coloring page – a family digitally communicating to a mental health provider.

Source: Perle, A. (2020). Children's coloring page - A family digitally communicating to a mental health provider [Unpublished drawing].

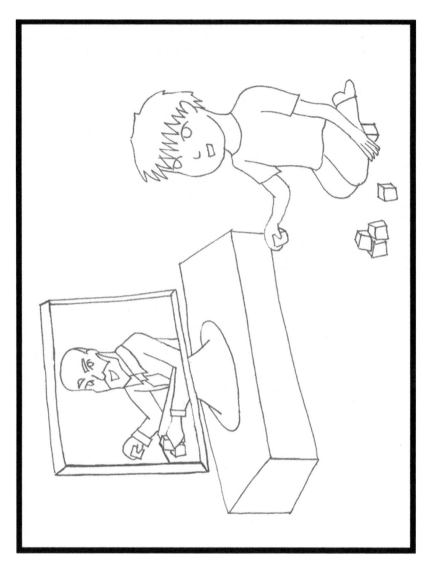

Figure K3 Children's coloring page – a child and mental health provider playing with blocks through videoconferencing.

Source: Perle, A. (2020). Children's coloring page - A child and mental health provider playing with blocks through videoconferencing [Unpublished drawing].

Appendix L: Preparing for Videoconferencing Patient Handout

Preparing for Videoconferencing Sessions

- I have high-speed/broadband internet.
- My provider and I agreed on the system that I will be using (e.g., computer, tablet, phone).
- My computer, tablet, or phone that I plan on using can run videoconferencing (e.g., it is a recent computer and has up-to-date software).
- My computer, tablet, or phone that I plan on using has an antivirus/antimalware program to ensure it is safe.
- I have a high-definition camera and microphone, and have tested them to make sure they work (e.g., newer video camera, newer laptop camera).
- I have a room (or rooms) specifically for the videoconferencing to make sure that it is as similar to visiting a provider's office as possible:
  - The room is private.
  - The room is quiet.
  - The room isn't cluttered or full of distractions.
  - I have tried to reduce interruptions (e.g., told others to not interrupt, put out "Do Not Disturb" sign).
  - I have placed the camera in a way so that the room is evenly lit (e.g., no windows or lighting directly behind me, which can cause shadowing).
  - I unplugged Alexa, Echo Dots, etc.
- Additional tips:
  - I will avoid wearing noisy clothing or jewelry.
  - I will avoid wearing bright, patterned, striped, checkered, or reflective clothing.
  - I will avoid wearing bright whites, reds, or oranges.
  - I will tell the provider if at any time I am having issues with my video or audio, or if the provider is hard to see or hear.
  - I will have my phone and/or email readily available during session in case the provider needs to get a hold of me.
  - If children will be present, avoid toys that create a lot of noise.

- I know how to troubleshoot the technology (e.g., computer, camera), if needed.
- I have spoken to my provider and understand what to do if the video-conferencing doesn't work:
  - Step 1: Attempt to restart the videoconferencing meeting or reboot internet connection.
  - Step 2: Lower the video or audio quality to create better connection, if possible.
  - Step 3: Try another videoconferencing method, as suggested by the provider.
  - Step 4: Use telephone for remainder of session, or reschedule, as indicated by the provider.

If you have questions or concerns about any of the above information, please contact your provider.

Index

For Product Safety Concerns and Information please contact our EU
representative GPSR@taylorandfrancis.com
Taylor & Francis Verlag GmbH, Kaufingerstraße 24, 80331 München, Germany

www.ingramcontent.com/pod-product-compliance
Ingram Content Group UK Ltd.
Pitfield, Milton Keynes, MK11 3LW, UK
UKHW021448080625
459435UK00012B/414